Praise for
A Soft Voice in
a Noisy World

"*Karl Robb's book offers sage advice and inspiration to help people affected by Parkinson's to LIVE with the disease. It is truly a guidebook for the Parkinson's journey, for those whose trip is just beginning as well as those who have traveled great distances with it.*"

—Jackie Hunt Christensen, author of *The First Year: Parkinson's Disease and Life with a Battery-operated Brain: A Patient's Guide to Deep Brain Stimulation for Parkinson's Disease*

"*I met Karl the year after he was officially diagnosed—he was the youngest person I had ever met with PD. This book is a "must read" for anyone who has been diagnosed with Parkinson's— care partners, family members, or friends. Karl offers wonderful, practical, common-sense ideas that apply to everyone no matter how long you have had this disease. However, of all these ideas/ suggestions the most important is Karl's attitude—and we could all learn from him.*"

—Carol Walton, Chief Executive Officer, The Parkinson Alliance

"Karl Robb's book draws you in to his life and makes the uninformed feel connected in a frank and true understanding of life with Parkinson disease. For all of the pain and challenges he has faced since his days as a young man dealing with this disease, his hope and optimism shows through in this book. As a Support Group leader for so many years he has impacted people's lives with his courage and honest approach. A Soft Voice in a Noisy World *allows you to see inside the real Karl Robb that we who know him have the pleasure of already experiencing. The path is not the story, the way Karl navigates the path is the real story."*

—Lou Nistler, Executive Director, Parkinson Foundation of the National Capital Area

"A Soft Voice in a Noisy World is a humble, insightful book about taking charge of one's life in the face of chronic illness. Karl Robb's proactive approach to battling Parkinson's is inspirational."

—Samantha Elandary, Founder and CEO, Parkinson Voice Project

A
Soft Voice
in a
Noisy World

A Guide to Dealing
and Healing with
Parkinson's Disease

A Soft Voice in a Noisy World

A Guide to Dealing
and Healing with
Parkinson's Disease

Karl Robb

RobbWorks
Fairfax, Virginia

Grateful acknowledgment is made for permission to reprint the article "Stress: How We Can Help Ourselves!" by Gilbert A. Gallego, which originally appeared in Parkinson Report, The Official Journal of the National Parkinson Foundation, vol. XVII, issue 4, Fall 2006. Copyright © 2006 by Gilbert A. Gallego.

Some of the material in this book was originally published in the blog ASoftVoice.com.

The information contained in this book is intended to provide helpful and informative material on the subjects addressed. It is not intended to serve as a replacement for professional medical, legal, or financial advice. Any use of the advice in this book is at the reader's discretion. The author and publisher specifically disclaim any and all liability arising directly or indirectly from the use or application of any information contained in this book. A health-care professional or attorney or financial advisor should be consulted regarding your specific situation. The intent of the author is to offer information of a general nature to help you in your quest for enhanced well-being. In the event you use any of the information in this book for yourself, the author and the publisher assume no responsibility for your actions.

RobbWorks books are available at quantity discounts for educational, business, or sales promotional use. For information, please email: bulksales@robbworks.com.

Publisher: RobbWorks
Email: asoftvoice@robbworks.com
Website: www.robbworks.com

Editing by Stephanie Gunning
Interior design by Gus Yoo
Cover design by Gus Yoo

ISBN 978-0-9881847-0-1 (paperback)
ISBN 978-0-9881847-1-8 (ebook)

1. Parkinson's disease 2. Reiki 3. Self-help 4. Chronic illness 5. Holistic health 6. Complementary therapies 7. Neurology

For Mom, who courageously battled cancer and motivated me to share my story.

Her inspiration made this book a reality.

For Angela, for her patience, strength, faith, and devotion.

I thank her for her love and selflessness in making my dreams hers.

I am eternally grateful that she is my best friend, wife, and partner.

Table of Contents

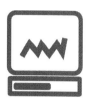

Foreword

Bill Moyers, award-winning broadcast journalist and author

This is a story of the hero's journey.

Not to outer space. Not to some distant battlefield. Not to glory on the athletic field. But to the most difficult of all places to sustain a struggle against the odds: to the inner reaches of one's own heart and mind, where the meaning of life is defined and the struggle ultimately won or lost.

In his classic book *The Hero with a Thousand Faces*, Joseph Campbell, who devoted his life to exploring themes of the world's great mythologies, defines the hero as a man or woman who has battled past limitations, beyond obstacles and seeming defeats, to seek and discover, in the primary springs of life, the power of transfiguration—and because of that journey to help others by sharing hard-won knowledge and wisdom.

Karl Robb is just such a hero. His is a remarkable personal journey with implications for all of us.

After several years of experiencing something amiss—bodily sensations that were puzzling and disconcerting but could not be pinpointed or identified by medical counsel—he was diagnosed at twenty-three with Parkinson's disease. There is no way an outsider like me can grasp what such a revelation must mean to someone so young, his adulthood opening before him, sprinting down-field like a fullback in the clear, on his way to a touchdown, only to be tackled from behind and brought forcefully and painfully to the ground.

I can only imagine the fear, bewilderment, and melancholy—above all, the anger—that would overwhelm anyone hearing the diagnosis: "Parkinson's disease." But in the early bloom of life? Young Robb knew no one even close to his age with the affliction. Hearing what lay ahead of him, the thought of losing control over his life had to leave him feeling cheated, alone, forlorn.

And yet he refused futility's embrace. For twenty years now he has made a fight of it, turning one difficult experience after enough into a continuing course in adult education for all of us—those who live with Parkinson's disease and those of us who barely know what the words mean. Karl would learn everything he could about the disease; he would plumb every source he could find; consult first one expert and then another, including the most informed experts of all, those living with the disease itself; try one treatment and then another, not only hoping that something better would come along but taking every initiative to turn that hope into reality. He found resources to cope, reasons to fight on, and strength to persist.

And now he has written this book—written it, I hasten to add, with the help of another hero of this story, his wife, Angela. The very title is as beguiling as the story is revealing: *"A Soft Voice in a Noisy World."* I have learned so much from that voice, and so will you. Whether you have Parkinson's disease or not, are a caregiver, or work in the health field, you will learn here about the disease, about hope and fear, about courage, the resolute heart—and even, I wager, about yourself. Because the message in these pages carries far beyond them: You, reader, have more power and control over your well-being than you know.

That, as Joseph Campbell told me in our PBS series on "The Power of Myth," is the ultimate discovery—and reward—of the hero's journey:

"People say that what we're all seeking is a meaning for life. I don't think that's what we're really seeking. I think that what we're seeking is an experience of being alive, so that our life experiences on the purely physical plane will have resonances within our innermost being and reality, so that we actually feel the rapture of being alive. That's what it's all finally about, and that's what these clues help us to find within ourselves."

Karl Robb shows us how under the most trying circumstances a human being can find strength and purpose beyond expectations. As he writes, "I have many purposes. I have a reason to heal for myself and those who care about me. My life has meaning and I will find strength and invigoration in everything I do from now on. Life has a new inspiration. A new challenge and I am willing to accept that challenge."

We are in Karl's debt for sharing with us his experience of being alive.

Bill Moyers

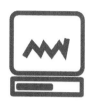

Foreword

Amy Comstock Rick, CEO, Parkinson's Action Network

I f you look up the word "advocate" in the dictionary, you'll see a photo of Karl Robb.

Advocacy has been a driving theme in Karl's life – whether it was struggling with doctors to be properly diagnosed with Parkinson's disease in his early twenties, managing the symptoms he experiences now, or fighting in Washington for federal funding toward better treatments and cure.

As CEO of the Parkinson's Action Network, of which Karl is a board member, I have seen first-hand how he not only manages his disease, but also thrives in advocacy and outreach to raise awareness. Along with his wife, Angela, Karl is an active voice in the fight for federal policy support for the Parkinson's community. He is always at the ready to go on Capitol Hill, in front of a television camera, or to meet with other advocates about how they can make a difference in their own health and for the Parkinson's community as a whole.

In this book, Karl poignantly shares his insights on what it's like to live with Parkinson's disease every day. But more than that, he writes about taking control. He shares ideas for activities people with Parkinson's – or most other diseases, really – can do to effect change in their own lives and the lives of others. Karl writes about remaining flexible, staying informed, and being inspired by both the little and big things around you. His advocacy work around quality of life issues for the Parkinson's community cannot go unnoticed. He motivates and inspires others with his experiences, and the community is all the better for it.

The Parkinson's disease community is comprised of so many people who are advocates for their own health, advocates for quality care for others, and advocates for research for ultimately finding a cure for this disease. Karl is a leader amongst that group and I am proud to have him as a friend. Karl, thank you for sharing your story.

Acknowledgments

I wrote this book for myself as much as for my friends seeking a way of understanding a life with Parkinson's disease. With their help, I've been able to find the strength within myself to accept and manage my condition. I believe that each of us has a valuable lesson to share with the rest of the world. What follows is a collection of my insights, epiphanies, wakeup calls, awakenings, and trial and error lessons. My intent in this book is to enlighten, inspire, teach, and entertain. It is my hope that you, the reader, feel encouraged to seek your path to health and wellness after reading this.

I want to thank my wife, Angela. Without her commitment to completing this book, it might have never made it out the door. Thank you for your love and support.

Thanks to my friends with and without Parkinson's disease, who have encouraged and supported me to get my story out.

Introduction

"It is common sense to take a method and try it. If it fails, admit it frankly and try another. But above all, try something."—Franklin D. Roosevelt

No one plans on being ill for most of his life. For some of us, however, illness is a dire reality of life. With time, awareness, and discovery, relief may come. Be it a medication, procedure, or therapy, those of us with chronic illness live in the hope of something better coming along to treat us and bring us relief. Our future is largely dependent upon the bureaucracy of the Food and Drug Administration (FDA), the National Institutes of Health (NIH), the drug companies, the medical community, and the federal government discovering and developing those new treatments. While we wait, there is still much more for us to discover.

Illness has a powerful influence on a young life. The insecurity of knowing that you are not completely well generates fear and questions about your mortality. My journey and many of my misadventures in seeking an answer to my medical frustrations are in this book. It is my intention that I can assist you in avoiding the mistakes that I made along this winding road.

I know of no illness that comes with a learning manual. I have written the manual that I wish I had received after finding out that I had Parkinson's disease (PD). I was only twenty-three when I got the diagnosis, but I knew something was amiss at least six years earlier.

Facing the issue of life or death and genuinely not having a clue about losing control of my body was frightening. At the time, there was no Internet and I didn't know anyone close to my age with PD. Most material that I could find was for much older patients. I felt totally isolated and unsure of my future. Knowing what I know now gives me hope and strength that as a young man weren't always there. I hope that my years of navigation bring you perspective and benefit.

I can say here and now that, after over twenty years of dealing with Parkinson's disease, I am seeing positive changes in my condition. I would even dare to say that "I see healing." It is my hope that you find a spark here in my manual for healing that you may add to your toolbox of health and wellness.

A Soft Voice in a Noisy World is a title with special meaning. A predominant number of people living with Parkinson's have difficulty being heard or understood because of their condition. While an individual may be soft spoken and not easily heard, the individual may still be thoughtful, cogent, and intelligent. Those who don't understand the symptoms of this disease may question that person's intellect because of the delivery of the message when really they would do better to base their impressions on the full content of the message being communicated.

People with Parkinson's disease, who are known as "Parkinsonians" or "Parkies," are often pre-judged by their movements, or lack thereof, their facial expressions, or lack thereof, and, ultimately, by their voices, or lack thereof. Outside factors, indirectly related to these individuals, can play a huge role in the severity of their condition: stress, diet, sleep, climate, and even something as innocuous as noise, can influence Parkinson's symptoms. The title reflects how the Parkinsonian's voice softens for some unknown reason. The voice is often unheard or lost in the din of daily life and the numerous distractions that come with it. Losing the voice can be one of the most devastating symptoms of Parkinson's.

Whether it is at a conference or at a support group meeting, I often hear my peers and their care partners—an appropriate term for the spouses and partners who help each other and share the care—ask for a list of what works for others in the group. This book is my compilation of what I find has improved life for me and for my care partner, Angela. As there is no user's manual *per se* for living with Parkinson's disease, I decided to write one.

Much of my philosophy and points on doctors and health transcend Parkinson's and would be applicable to living with any kind of chronic illness. Sadly, the possibility exists for any of us to get sick. No one is immune. I believe that the chronically ill have a special insight and an appreciation for life that may get lost by those not afflicted.

Time is our worst enemy and yet our best friend at the same time. Parkinson's disease affects us all so differently and at such different rates that there is no telling how fast it might progress. We must wait patiently for a scientific breakthrough. Time is our friend because we are living and here. As long as we are here, we have options and the opportunity to seek out a solution to our problems. Those not familiar with this illness or dealing with any illness are incapable of totally understanding what it is to live ill. Whether you're living with chronic illness, are caring for someone struggling with a chronic illness, are employed in the healthcare field, or you are just looking to get a patient's perspective on dealing with and living with an illness, the intention of this book is to provide you with a fresh outlook on illness, and a plan for improving the quality of your life and preparing for the later stages of your illness.

More than half of my life has been spent navigating the world of medicine and doctors. Since my diagnosis with Parkinson's disease at age twenty-three, I have been active in the Parkinson's community. Through advocacy work with the Parkinson's Action Network (PAN) and assisting in numerous conferences for the National Parkinson Foundation (NPF), I have made lasting friendships with an incredible network of people with Parkinson's who have inspired me to get my story out.

It is my sincere wish that this book makes a positive and lasting change in your life. May this book help lead you on your path to health and healing. With love and compassion, I wish you the best. If you get only one thing out of this book, in my view, it should be the understanding that you have more power and control over your well-being than you know. From your choice of the drugs you take, to the foods you eat and the doctors who advise your progress, you are in charge. You are your own best advocate.

My journey is far from over and I am still learning and discovering. Finding answers and solving problems with unconventional methods may take a bit of a mind shift. Each of us has our own unique journey to follow as we move along our path to healing.

Finding relief from illness requires investigation, research, and devotion. Only through tenacious and vigorous exploration will you ultimately find the solutions you need to manage your symptoms. It may take vitamins, complementary therapies, medications, meditation, exercise, hypnosis, or something completely foreign to you. My introduction to Reiki, a type of energy therapy, almost fourteen years ago, led me on my path to health and healing. It changed my life for the better. We are all unique and mysterious puzzles. We Parkinsonians are the ambassadors for Parkinson's disease. It is our right, responsibility, and duty to make a difference for ourselves and for all those with Parkinson's who are unable to be heard and are seeking a better way of life.

How to Use This Book

Illness doesn't come with a manual. In my over twenty-year history with Parkinson's disease, I have searched for a guide to positive living and helpful tools. I wanted insights and helpful information that I could use to help myself. The information is out there, but it took me all this time to compile and gain the knowledge to lead me down the path of healing and wellness. I have come a long way and I promise you that something in this book will hit a chord with you.

It is my sincere hope that you or the person you care about is able to open this book to any page and find something informative and useful.

Feel free to start at any page. It's up to you how you use this book. I wish you a journey of healing experiences and finding what you seek along the way.

The Pledge of the Ill

Before reading further, I invite you to take the following pledge.

I accept my illness, but it does not define me. I am so much more, even if my illness masks or prohibits others from seeing who I am. Though I am different, I reserve the right to receive patience, respect, and some level of understanding from those I encounter in my everyday life.

I acknowledge that I have a duty to myself to explore all potential modes of healing whether they are conventional or out of the mainstream. I am worthy of being cared for by medical practitioners who treat me with respect and are willing to listen to me. I deserve to be recognized by my physician or other healthcare provider as a person with a life, not just as someone with a medical problem and a chart. My physician owes me the understanding to speak with me as an equal and as a human being, making my way through life as best as I possibly can.

I am willing to make changes, adjustments, and even sacrifices of monumental proportion if these therapies will assist in my betterment and the betterment of the lives of those around me. I am a representative of all those others, before and yet to follow me, who are afflicted with my very same illness. I will do all that I can for myself and those who are similarly afflicted.

I am on a journey to health and healing. I will share my insights and take time to educate all who will listen to me about my disease. The world needs more compassion, and only through education and understanding can we gain true compassion. I don't need, want, or desire any kind of sympathy, because sympathy is far too close to pity. All I ask for is assistance in moving along my path to achieve, learn, teach, grow, and inspire.

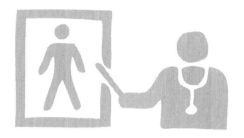

PART ONE

If Doctors Had All the Answers, Medicine Wouldn't Be Called a "Practice"

CHAPTER 1
Prelude to a Diagnosis

"No man is a good doctor who has never been sick himself."—Chinese proverb

The onset of Parkinson's disease was gradual, but steady—although I had no real idea of what was happening to me. At seventeen, I experienced intermittent episodes wherein my knee, foot, or hand would shake. Slowly, my speech became more broken. My body became stiffer and I felt less flexible. I began to slouch in my chair. My handwriting got smaller and harder to read. I noticed I was dragging my feet and the length of my stride shortened. Over time, my arms would fail to keep in sync with my legs when I walked. Sometimes, my arms didn't move with my legs at all.

I was well enough to continue pursuing the routines of a youthful life. I had graduated with decent grades from high school and spent a year on the tennis team. After two years at the University of Georgia, I transferred back to my native North Carolina and the University of North Carolina at Chapel Hill to complete my degree in English.

College was a challenge. My body was letting me down more often. From my walking to my talking, I was observing a distinct change. I'm sure many of my fellow classmates considered me to be strange as a result of how I moved and spoke. Dating was difficult because I appeared awkward and unpolished. This was hard for a young man who had always admired James Bond and hoped to achieve "cool" someday.

I didn't understand what was happening to my body. I wanted answers. My search, however, would stall out temporarily after going to the Student Health Center and to a top medical school hoping for a diagnosis only to be told, "It is just stress. Chill out and have a beer!" Retrospectively, it is evident this was not the advice I needed.

While I did all right in college, I wasn't able to enjoy it as fully as I had hoped. Even so, I was able to learn more about my identity and the person I hoped to become.

Following my graduation, I experienced one of the most humiliating and yet enlightening moments of my life. I believe that this may have been my first realization that I had a serious problem. My father, feeling that I needed to face and overcome a challenge in order to build my confidence, strongly suggested I look into Outward Bound, a wilderness program that my elder brother had completed many years earlier. All I could remember my brother saying about the program afterwards was how each night the participants would sit around and "express their inner feelings." I had a little clearer picture of what to expect after I read the Outward Bound promotional brochure, but I had no idea just how far over my head I was going to be.

For three months, I worked out three or four days a week to build up my strength in preparation for what sounded like a demanding and rigorous, yet doable, mountain experience. When I jogged in the park, I sometimes actually had to run into a tree and wrap my arms around it to break the built-up momentum. To this day, I am amazed that I didn't get more stares than I did from people on the street. Something was happening, but we failed to see the signs.

After these few months of breaking in boots, hand-picking each piece of camping gear, and toning my body to what I thought was tiptop shape, I felt I was ready. Nothing could have prepared me adequately for the events of the next five days.

It was late June in the Blue Ridge Mountains of Western North Carolina. This area is one of the most unpredictable parts of the state to forecast weather due to the varying winds and fronts that cross these mountains. The standard joke is: "If you don't like the weather, wait five minutes." Up there it's not a joke. Mother Nature plays the gamut. Unlike most of the Southeast, the North Carolina mountains generally provide some relief from the oppressive summer humidity, and it is usually ten to fifteen degrees cooler there than in most of the state. This summer was more unpredictable than most. Not only would the next few weeks be excessively humid, they would set new rainfall records as well.

It was four o'clock and our Outward Bound group had assembled in a parking lot at the bottom of Grandfather Mountain. I was eager to hike the trails and see wildlife. I had no idea just how difficult some of our hikes (night and day) and river crossings would be.

The afternoon was gray, cold, and windy—gusts had to be nearly fifty miles an hour—with a light rain. The trail was strenuous, and with our packs it seemed damned near impossible. When we approached the exposed face of the mountain, I had a strong feeling that not only was I very close to nature, but also very close to death. Grandfather Mountain has recorded some of the highest winds of any place in the United States, with winds measuring as high as 200 miles per hour. My group had left the trail and we were now climbing a slick, wet rock face about 5,000 feet above sea level. One slip and any of us easily could have fallen to our death. The driving wind and rain worsened. There was no sign of it letting up. We made camp and put up our tarps and unpacked our gear.

Outward Bound promotes low-impact camping, the aim of which is to try and leave Nature as you find it. Rather than using a tent, everyone found a place beneath a piece of plastic stretched between two trees. In a torrential downpour, a tarp won't keep you dry. Throughout the night, water trickled off my tarp and down into my sleeping bag. Even so, I fell asleep and slept straight through until morning. When you are completely exhausted, it is shocking what you can sleep through.

On day two, the rain continued. By now we were all carrying at least an extra ten pounds of water in our packs. Not one item any of us had was dry. Everything we possessed was drenched. The summer humidity didn't let up. The heat and humidity brought out more biting insects than I had ever seen. The trails had begun to soften and wash away, only to reveal mud, rocks, and tree roots. Some of the washouts created narrow canals, leaving us no convenient place to step with our waterlogged boots. Frequently, if a path was too slick and steep, we were able to straddle the ditch with a foot on either side. Moving was slow and tiring. We were all tired, soaked, and hungry. Straddling became nearly impossible when we reached the steep inclines and long descents. The washed out paths made secure footing a challenge of balance and stamina. Although it was certainly difficult for the others, too, it was even more difficult for me than for them because of my stiffening muscles, mild tremor, and lack of speed.

That afternoon, one of our group members had a frightening misfortune. He caught his foot on a protruding root, causing him to fall head over heels and hit his head. Blood trickled from his ear and he got cold quickly. One of the staff had an emergency radio and called for assistance. Miles from any kind of help or civilization, two of our guides left us to rush the injured man to get medical attention. The rest of the group moved on. We never saw him again.

On our third day out, late in the afternoon, the group was encamped up on a ridge. Almost instantly, we were engulfed in a lightning storm.

We were instructed to rush to the lowest part of the ridge with our packs and told to sit on top of them in order to avoid having any contact with the rocky ground, as rock conducts electricity. Within a matter of minutes, the lightning was right on top of us. North Carolina is one of the top states for frequent lightning strikes. While stuck up on the ridge, lightning struck. One of my friends, Mike, received a shot of ground current during that storm. To my amazement, he was only stunned briefly and showed no wear from the power surge.

Given my physical limitations, which included a strange phenomenon of sudden forward propelling (festination), and my general shakiness and inflexibility, I thought I was handling myself adequately. I was thankful that whenever I slowed down or my knee locked on me during stream crossings Mike was there to help and encourage me. As my legs continued to stiffen and my hands and feet shook at times, my friends and the staff began to worry about me. After experiencing the aforementioned moments of terror and exhilaration with my newfound friends, my group leaders told me that I could no longer be part of this group because I posed a "health risk both to myself and to the members of the group." First, they told me that they would put the subject of my continuation of the trip to a group decision. If my peers felt that I was a burden, then they would let me go. But, when not even one group member wanted me to leave, the instructors still said I had to go, anyhow. Their decision was devastating to me. A bond had been built between me and the others and now they were being stripped from me for no understandable fault of my own.

My drive to prove myself and my denial that anything was wrong was potentially a danger to the other members of the group, yet I was unable to see this at the time. In my mind, I wanted to complete this program and nothing was going to stop me. I didn't know why I trembled when it wasn't cold or why my knees locked up on me in river crossings or why my momentum constantly propelled me forward. All I knew was that I had set out to complete this wilderness course. I had made some great new friends, but my unknown ailment was scaring these instructors, and me. An instructor was tasked with taking me back to base camp.

We were about twelve miles from any signs of civilization. We hiked about eight miles until we came to a dirt road where we hitched a ride from a passing pickup truck. We got out at an old general store like the ones you see in the movies. From there the instructor called for Outward Bound to send a driver to come and get us and take us to base camp. I was being treated like I was having a medical emergency. I was dazed and confused. I felt dejected and cast out. This wasn't what I had wanted or expected. Now, one journey was over and it was time for a new one to begin.

When the car arrived to pick us up, I remember the driver got out of the car, came around to the other side, opened my door for me, took my pack from me, and spoke very slowly and childlike, as if I were incapable of understanding what was happening. I had showed muscular problems, not mental problems, as far as I could tell, yet I was being treated like a child. All I could think was that things were changing, and not in a direction that I had anticipated.

Back at Outward Bound base camp, I was treated differently than the other participants. I noticed that the instructors spoke more deliberately to me and tried to cater to my needs a little too much. There was a sympathetic tone in their voices that seemed unnatural. I had apparently become the "weird guy."

The instructors told me that they had called my parents who would come pick me up in the morning. That night, I was to have dinner with a graduating class that had completed another nine-day mountain intensive course. For all intents and purposes, I had completed the same program as those guys, yet I didn't see the accomplishment. I felt defeated and out of place.

At dinner they made a toast recognizing me as someone sent back due to medical reasons, so I ended up needing to explain what that meant to an ongoing string of different curious individuals at intervals throughout the dinner. At least thirty well-meaning Outward Bound grads came across the room to introduce themselves, wish me well, and find out what my story was. I know they all meant well. These people felt sorry for me and, for the first time in my life, I was feeling sorry for myself and I wasn't sure why. I think I was missing my friends and I didn't want to give up on the trip. All I knew was that I never wanted to feel that way again.

For the next few days, I faced my first and only bouts of depression and anxiety about my con-

Prelude to a Diagnosis

dition. My self-esteem was as low as it had ever been. I was ashamed of myself for being thrown out of Outward Bound. My parents understood that it wasn't my fault and when I called my friends who expected me to still be hiking, they too understood and accepted that things like this happen and it really wasn't a big deal. The reality of the situation was a hard one to face. Looking back, I think it was a turning point in my life. I needed answers.

If you're wondering now why I had felt compelled to do Outward Bound, remember that there was a point to doing the program. Even though I was consistently wet, tired, hungry, sore, blistered, bug bitten, and frustrated with my body, I felt a strong connection with Nature. It felt right. It felt powerful. I had set out to complete a challenge. I was doing it to boost my confidence and prove my resilience just like everyone else who does it. Sadly, the outcome had temporarily backfired. Now I was worried about my well-being. No one could give me a real solution to what was happening with my body. I was getting concerned and needed answers.

I think I proved to myself what I needed to prove without completing the program. Maybe. Maybe not. The truth was that I'm not like everyone else, and I had to learn to accept that reality. As a person with Parkinson's disease, I have to accept this fact on a daily basis. There is nothing wrong with being different. We are all different, through no fault of our own. Everyone has limitations that they hit at some point. Unless you push your limits, you won't know where they are.

Whatever I had was growing slowly, and progressively worse. Something needed to be done. Back at home, I made an appointment to see a physician who was the chief motion specialist at a prestigious southern medical school. Not knowing anything about the disease except its name, I took a stab in the dark and asked if he thought my condition might be Parkinson's disease. I'll never forget his reply, because he was so mistaken, despite his credentials. "You're far too young to get Parkinson's disease," he said. "People your age just don't get Parkinson's disease. Chill out—have a beer!" This was medical advice? I thought. "There have been a few rare cases of people under fifty-five getting Parkinson's, but you don't have the symptoms."

I didn't have the symptoms? I lacked the classic habit of pill rolling and the "face masking," or expressionlessness, that Parkinsonians typically develop. This doctor wouldn't even consider there to be a chance of PD. I left his office with some useless medication for Benign Essential Tremor (BET). The meds did nothing and the doctor had no answers.

My expulsion from the program at the time made me feel angry, embarrassed, and rejected. There had been a week or more where I felt almost no sense of accomplishment afterward and stubbornly refused to consider that I might have a health problem. I wasn't willing to accept the facts, yet. Deep down, I had the terrible fear that I had brain cancer or some sort of unfound tumor.

I've met people who endured batteries of tests over long periods of time only to find no comfort in receiving a diagnosis. These are the people to feel for, not me. I truly believe that not knowing what you have is worse than getting a scary diagnosis. I was prepared to receive news of multiple sclerosis or brain cancer. Not knowing what I had was incredibly frustrating.

It took a while, but seven months after my Outward Bound trip, after seeing six or more doctors, and six years from my earliest recognized symptoms, I would finally get an accurate diagnosis.

CHAPTER 2
The Diagnosis

"Drugs are not always necessary. Belief in recovery always is."—Norman Cousins

I had hoped that Outward Bound would give me some insight on what would come next in my life. It took me down an unexpected path, but it did help me to see what I had to do. While searching for answers, I had to do something. I decided with my dad that I would move to Colorado for the winter while I was seeking a diagnosis.

My symptoms had worsened and I'd reached the point to where I was walking bent over like a hunchback. My gait was rigid and my knees were constantly flexed. When I walked or attempted to walk, because of my stiffness in my lower body, the forward momentum of my upper body, a symptom called "festination," would propel my body forward and be forced to run into fixed objects to break the momentum. Mailboxes, lamp posts, and telephone poles became my best friends. I must have looked bizarre as I clung to these objects for stability.

More than once, I was asked if I was drunk or under the influence of some substance. The staggered walk and broken speech definitely are attributes of PD that resemble inebriation. When it was convenient and I didn't want to tell my story, I'd laugh and say that I had a little too much, even though I've never been an excessive drinker. Sometimes, I would use the excuse that I was working out. Looking back, the frustration and an embarrassment that I felt from these public PD symptoms was wasted energy. I created added stress for no fault of my own.

Had I known then, what I know now, the whole situation would have been different. I might have been more honest about it. I wasn't ready to explain myself or admit to others just what was happening to me. I wasn't even sure myself. I avoided going out because I could barely walk, and if I could walk, I trembled—and I was tired of using the "caffeine overdose" excuse. Thinking back, I regret the lies. I also forgive myself for them, because at that time I had no real explanation. Of course, the doctors I consulted didn't have any answers for me either.

I hope that your physician has a good bedside manner. Many of my earlier doctors had minimal people skills. If you're a doctor, this may be hard for you to hear. I hope you take these words to heart. Not one of the doctors that I had seen thus far—there were at least five of them—had really taken the time to talk to me as a human being.

They had merely treated me as an intriguing case study and lab experiment, an anomaly, or a personal challenge.

For myself, I was concerned and highly motivated to pursue an answer. I wasn't scared. I was curious. I just needed to know why my body was turning against me and how to stop it. I had to know how serious my condition truly was.

I went to see Dr. 6, who referred me to Dr. 7, a neurologist. Although a supposedly fine neurologist himself, Dr. 6 wasn't willing to make the diagnosis, so he referred me to this other neurologist who specialized in treating children and young people. Dr. 7, the juvenile medicine expert from New York, was to join the practice the following week and it was suggested that I come back then after they had discussed my case.

Following a barrage of more tests and questions by Dr. 7, I was hopeful that this wasn't another dead end. However, this time the whole process was tenser and a little more frustrating than it previously had been. In addition to the tests of my bodily fluids and observations of my movement that I'd become accustomed to, I now underwent a magnetic resonance imaging scan (MRI) to check my brain for heavy metals, tumors, and anomalies . If you're not familiar with the MRI machine, it's something like a round, space age-designed coffin that takes pictures of your insides. (Since the twentieth century, when it first came into use, MRI technology has progressed and there are more options.)

As a borderline claustrophobe, I found spending an hour in the MRI to be a very uncomfortable experience. The process itself is painless, but anyone with a fear of confining spaces can find it more than unnerving. One friend of mine couldn't stay inside for the entire period. Surprisingly, I endured the test from beginning to end. Due to my deteriorating gait, stuttering speech, and occasional tremor, in the back of my mind I was sure that I had a brain tumor. In my mind, none of these symptoms made sense. I was young and relatively healthy in spite of my neurological system.

It was a Friday afternoon at four. Dr. 7 had promised to call me then with the results of my MRI and blood work, and to report back with a diagnosis after reviewing my medical history. He had alluded to the possibility of Parkinson's disease, but was not willing to make a definitive diagnosis until all the information came back. I was in agony from waiting.

My father phoned the doctor's office at the appointed time on my behalf and found out that the doctor's office was doctor-less. A nurse, lacking any smidgen of tact, told my father matter-of-factly, "We're treating him for Parkinson's disease." This was to be my confirmation? Where was the professionalism...the tact...the understanding? What if my diagnosis had been a fatal, inoperable brain tumor—is that how I would have found out? My parents and I were stunned, vexed, and perplexed that any doctor or nurse would deliver such a staggering, life-changing diagnosis in such a cold and compassionless manner as I had received mine. The weekend was full of questions with no answers. As this was prior to the Internet, easy information access was not available.

While the diagnosis was a shock at first and then a mystery, the diagnosis itself came as a massive relief. I had gone so long without a diagnosis and an answer to what exactly I was facing that the diagnosis gave me peace. It was good news that I wasn't going to die of a terminal brain tumor in six months as I had envisioned. At least for the time being, my inexplicable symptoms could be explained. The disease had a name and I had a prognosis. The hardest part of dealing with illness is fighting an unknown enemy. How do you battle an enemy you've never encountered before and don't know? How do you fight a disease that isn't named and fully categorized? Knowing your enemy is a crucial component to winning the battle and ultimately the war.

I had forced myself to prepare for the inevitable end of my life to come very soon. Now that I knew I would live (and once I got over being mad at how the news was so insensitively delivered) I could start to break down the problems and figure out what my options were.

When we finally connected directly with the doctor, we found out from him that the results which came back showed nothing really out of whack. PD is a disease without an easy and definite diagnosis to confirm the onset. It is a symptomatic disease. For many patients, the only way to confirm PD is after an autopsy, and I felt that might be a little premature in my case. Normally, if a patient shows signs of three or more symptoms of PD, then they will be diagnosed with "Parkinsonism." Looking back, I had one of the classic early-onset symptoms: constipation. Constipation can be a precursor to Parkinson's, which can crop up years before a motor symptom arises. Another symptom that often shows up early is the loss of the ability to smell certain odors. I may have had that but I'm not sure. Dr. 7 and his team decided that I should experiment with a medication called Sinemet to see if it would relieve my symptoms. Ever since then, Sinemet, the gold standard drug for PD, has been one of the keys to keeping me active and alert much of the time.

Within twenty-four hours and after taking three doses of Sinemet, a miracle seemed to occur. The symptoms that had been plaguing me subsided. A dramatic transformation took place. Now, I was walking with full arm swings and a gait reminiscent of an athletic ability that hadn't been there for years. My movements were fluid. My back straightened, my knees unlocked, and the overall rigidity in my body was gone. I was overjoyed, as were my parents. The muscular control that had escaped me so gradually returned in just a matter of hours.

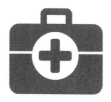

CHAPTER 3
Frustrations with Doctors

Some live their lives on Standard Time.
Others follow Greenwich Mean Time.
The free and easy follow Island Time.
But the unpredictable prescribe to PD Time.

Never knowing, Will my meds work?
Will my body do as I ask of it?
Must I wait and postpone my plans?
PD Time dominates my life and the life of my care
  partner.

I had come a long way. I was standing more erect, I was swinging my arms when I walked, and my gait was much improved. My disease had been diagnosed and effectively treated to the point where my noticeable symptoms were apparently being managed. Not knowing much about Parkinson disease, I was curious. I immediately began to read books and newsletters on PD. I even decided to attend the next convention of the American Parkinson's Disease Association.

My doctor told me that during the first week of treatment I would remain on a dosage of three pills a day of Sinemet. After six weeks I was expected to move up to eight pills a day. But I was soon to learn what it is to have too much of a good thing. After only a few days, I experienced violent twisting of my upper torso and extreme restlessness in my hands, shoulders, and feet. I'd already read accounts of this side effect, but figured it was only caused by much larger doses. Not knowing enough about PD or my medication, I searched for an answer with the help of friends. A good friend of my family led me to a gentleman named Leon Sack, who not only had PD, but also published a Parkinson's disease newsletter.

I called Mr. Sack and spoke to him for close to an hour. After my description of how my hands would fight one another as they gripped the steering wheel when I drove, Mr. Sack shared similar experiences with this frustrating and potentially dangerous side effect. He said that I was probably taking too much medication and that the drug might be causing *dyskinesia*, a side effect that occurs when the body gets too much dopamine. This troubling side effect can be more of a problem than the disease itself. I obviously needed to lower my dose.

When I told Mr. Sack about the program my doctors had prescribed of rapidly moving up my dosage to eight pills within six weeks, he gave me the name of his own doctor, whom I would later learn was one of the leading experts in the field, William C. Koller, M.D., Ph.D., Professor and Chairman of Neurology at University of Kansas Medical Center, Kansas City, Kansas. I remember the first time I spoke with Dr. Koller. He returned my phone call within the hour and he expressed a great deal of interest in me. He helped me sort out the issue of my Sinemet dosage with Dr. 7. With Dr. Koller's help, I was able to remain on a low dosage of Sinemet.

I sometimes think how my nervous system might have been shattered if I had stayed on the program Dr. 7 laid out for me. To increase up to eight pills in six weeks could have been devastating to my system. Over twenty years later, I am on a lower dosage than when I began the Sinemet. I am convinced that had I remained on Dr. 7's scale-up on Sinemet I would have over stimulated my neurons and my body! I know for sure that I would have been bouncing off the walls with uncontrollable energy.

A Parkinsonian experiencing dyskinesia may find it nearly impossible to do any kind of normal daily activity whether it's trying to bring a glass to your mouth, typing a letter, or something as simple as signing your name. Dyskinesia can be frustrating and debilitating.

My doctor, Dr. 7, met a doctor at a conference and suggested I go see this doctor in Chicago to confirm his own diagnosis of me. I was told that this guy was an expert in the field. Not until I arrived, however, did I find out that Dr. 8 was actually an expert in multiple sclerosis (MS), rather than Parkinson's. My brother, Richard, who was living in Chicago, kindly gave me a place to crash and agreed to accompany me to the new doctor's office.

Dr. 7 in Charlotte had overnighted the file containing the results of my numerous tests, blood work, and MRI sheets two weeks ahead of my visit to meet this expert, Dr. 8. Richard and I went to the hospital to meet Dr. 8. After waiting almost four hours, we were called in by a medical intern who asked many of the basic questions that go with a first visit. Amazingly, she had no record that my doctor in Charlotte had set up this appointment. She didn't even know why I was there. An hour later, the doctor himself walked in. The first thing I remember him saying was, "How can I help you today?"

Frankly, I was flabbergasted. I had left my job in Colorado and flown in to Chicago to get a confirmation of my diagnosis from someone who had no background on me. We asked him if he had looked at my file, to which he replied, "What file?" We were now five hours into our hospital visit.

After a half hour of searching, Dr. 8 and his staff found the file. He showed only a vague recollection of meeting Dr. 7, and their relationship was clearly only a minimal association. We watched him looking at my file for an uncomfortable five minutes. When he had glanced through most of the file, he remarked, "Well, it looks like you have Parkinson's disease," and laughed.

Had I really flown all that distance just to hear him say this? Not a chance. If the diagnosis needed confirming, we wanted him to confirm it. My brother and I pitched a number of suggestions of alternative diseases at Dr. 8 other than PD, to see what he thought. Maybe this was a mistake because I was set up for a new battery of tests after our pitch session. The doctor's staff took twelve vials of blood from my arm, gave me a urine test and an electric response test, and then finally did a lumbar puncture to take some spinal fluid.

After giving me the spinal tap, the doctor wanted me to stay in the hospital overnight, but I had been there all day and really wanted to leave. First, I hate hospitals. Second, I knew it was going to be way too expensive. Third, the last place I wanted to be was in an unfamiliar city and in a hospital bed. I talked him out of making me stay overnight and went home with Richard.

I returned to Colorado and awaited my final results. That particular wait never ended. The doctor in Chicago was far from cooperative in getting me results of the many tests I had taken—though his bills were right on time, and plentiful. I got numerous calls from the Chicago hospital asking me why I hadn't paid and in reply I asked, "Where are the test results that I'm paying for?" They never had a good answer to my question.

Weeks later, I found out from Dr. 7 in Charlotte that another colleague of his at Duke University Hospital was interested in doing exploratory surgery to test my arterial gases and biopsy my stomach. I questioned this suspicious surgery and asked my doctor about its expense and his reason for recommending this procedure. Apparently, I was a medical wonder. My doctor's colleague wanted to document me with an experimental investigative surgery that I was supposed to pay for. I asked Dr. 7, "What is he searching for?" and the answer was, "He is searching for a disease with no name and no symptoms."

Not a big fan of unnecessary surgery, I declined the generous offer and began my search for new medical counsel to help me manage my Parkinson's symptoms going forward.

By the time I flew out to Kansas City to meet Dr. Koller months later, I knew I had found the right doctor for me. Unlike the staff who worked for Dr. 8 in Chicago, who kept me waiting for the "great man" for hours, Dr. Koller's nurse called me in earlier than my appointment. Not only was she thoroughly friendly and personable, she listened well. When the doctor arrived, he also took the time to hear my medical stories as well as my personal ones. He answered all my questions and took the time I needed without making me feel rushed. This was the first time in my life that I could say I enjoyed going to see my doctor.

Bill Koller became a friend of mine and was a valuable resource to me in learning to live with Parkinson's. Had I not had access to him when I did, the consequences to my future health could have been devastating. I am eternally grateful to him for his life-saving aid and friendship. He is gone now and I miss him. I have yet to meet anyone else quite like him. He left us far too early.

Had Dr. Koller not introduced me to Dr. Linda Sigmund, my neurologist for the past fifteen years, I don't know what I would have done. Through mutual respect and sharing the understanding that I know my body and the medication, we have always been able to tweak the medication to fit my symptoms, together.

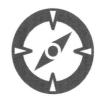

CHAPTER 4
Finding the Right New Doctor

"We are always paid for our suspicion by finding what we suspect."—Henry David Thoreau

Two of the most important decisions you will make as a Parkinsonian are your selections of a general practitioner and a neurologist. Here are four ways to find excellent doctors.

First, consult the members of your local Parkinson's disease support group and ask for their referrals to good doctors. You'll hear from patients who are satisfied and patients who are dissatisfied in these groups. Ask those who are happy or unhappy, "Why?"

Second, research your candidate doctors on the Internet. Start on Google, Yahoo!, and the other search engines. See if any red flag warnings come up. Read the websites of their practices. Compare and contrast the credentials of candidates.

Third, when selecting a general practitioner, ask if the doctor understands Parkinson's disease and the potential dangers of medications, combinations of medications, and certain types of surgeries.

Fourth, when selecting a neurologist, ask if this doctor is a movement disorders specialist. If you have early-onset Parkinson's disease, like I do, seeking a doctor with this credential is particularly meaningful to you. You will want a general practitioner and a neurologist who will compare notes to keep an eye on your condition.

These are just a few tips I hope that will help. You can also contact the different foundations and associations for individuals with Parkinson's disease and their families. See the Recommended Resources section at the back of the book for a list.

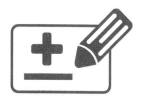

CHAPTER 5
Is Your Current Doctor Satisfactory?

A good fighter needs a good team behind him.

While your doctor is your connection to traditional medicine, keep an open mind to complementary therapies and options such as massage, yoga, Reiki, and other practices, changes in diet and exercise, as these may lead to potential relief from your condition. It is critical that you take charge of your body. Your healing begins and ends with you. Knowledge is power. Empower yourself with as much information as you can absorb. Many of the websites available on the Internet for Parkinsonians are full of valuable, up-to-date information and resources that you will want to share with your healthcare practitioner. Do be aware, there is plenty of misleading information to weed out as well. I have included a Resources section at the back of the book for your consideration.

It is extremely important that you and your doctor have a plan for your disease that you both can agree upon. If you feel your doctor isn't listening to your needs or is unwilling to take your best interests to heart, you may need to explore finding another doctor. This is your life, so you must look out for yourself as you try to maneuver through the minefield of the healthcare system.

Your doctor will be one of the many keys you need to manage a life with PD. If your doctor causes you frustration and anxiety, that's something you just don't need. You are entitled to have access to a health practitioner who cares about you and can aid you in your daily journey with your condition. If you aren't getting the service and treatment that you feel you deserve, say something (if appropriate) or just go out and identify a replacement doctor who can meet your needs better. It's okay to change doctors for personality reasons, too. Sadly, not all insurance plans allow for this kind of flexibility. Going to the doctor really shouldn't have to be an experience you dread.

Answer the following yes/no questions to determine if your doctor is right for you. Remember, your doctor works for you. Don't let him/her intimidate you!

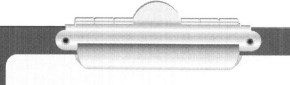

Are You Happy with Your Doctor?

• Is your doctor up to speed on new developments in your field of need? Y/N

• Does your doctor return your phone calls on a timely basis? Y/N

• Is your doctor usually on time? Y/N

• Is the doctor's office accommodating in helping you get your medications and refills when you need them? Y/N

• Does your doctor seem to care about your condition? Y/N

• Does your doctor have an open mind about holistic and complementary medicines and therapies? Y/N

• How is your doctor's bedside manner? Satisfactory/Unsatisfactory

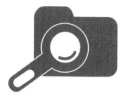

CHAPTER 6
Getting a Second Opinion

When it involves your health, seek peace of mind.

'd been watching television on a Sunday afternoon when my heart started racing uncontrollably. My mind was frantic. My body felt totally out of sync. I was frightened because my breathing seemed difficult. When I could finally force my mind to calm down sufficiently, I proceeded to meditate, and the frenetic slideshow of images in my brain and the rapid pulsations in my heart slowed, temporarily. This was the most difficult meditation that I can ever remember doing.

Amazingly, when I experience dyskinesia I can pull my mind and body back under some semblance of control through the use of meditation and Reiki. I had never felt this out of control. It was as if my mind and heart had lost contact with each other. In this instance, I honestly didn't know if I was experiencing a heart attack. I was getting frightened. It had to be happening on a Sunday of all days.

I considered going to the emergency room and rejected the idea because frequently doctors in the emergency room are unaware of, or are unfamiliar with the complexities of the Parkinsonian. I've heard numerous stories about patients entering the hospital only to receive their medicines late or even getting unnecessary treatment. My understanding of hospitals is that many don't usually let you take your meds on your own schedule; instead you are forced to surrender your meds so that they can distribute them to you. Every Parkinsonian knows from being on a schedule of medication that he or she needs their meds on time. I didn't want to lose control of my meds. Timing your medications right is a crucial part of living well with Parkinson's.

Though it was a weekend, I called my general practitioner, who told me to come in on Monday to be seen by his in-house cardiologist. I had no history of heart problems. I was young, active, and had eaten a vegetarian diet most of my life. While I was worried, I really didn't expect the cardiologist to find anything out of the ordinary.

The cardiologist was a grandfatherly gentleman whom I thought understood that I had Parkinson's. After giving my heart a listen and a cursory echocardiogram (EKG), Dr. Grandpa said it looked fine, but he suggested I come back a week later and do a stress test to be sure. He was nice enough, but seemed uncomfortable and distracted. I was nervous and he did little to ease the tension.

Protein can alter the effectiveness of the drugs that Parkinsonians take. Throughout the day you may be performing great one minute and then find that the medicine just isn't working the next. This is the curse that can accompany PD. You'll never know when to expect it, but at some point your meds may simply "turn off." That's what happened to me on the day of the stress test.

I got to the doctor's office early, arriving around 2:30 p.m. for the 3:00 p.m. appointment. I had eaten little that day in an effort to keep my protein intake down, and then was kept waiting almost an hour before the nurses prepped me for the stress test. Another twenty-five minutes went by as I lay shirtless on the icy metal table in the exam room. My hands and feet were turning a deep red and feeling icy cold. When the doctor finally strolled in as if nothing was wrong, I could tell my meds were turning off. The frustration of this encounter wasn't helping the situation either.

The demeanor of the cardiologist was less than cordial. He spoke to me and my wife as if we didn't understand English. He wasn't apologetic about confining us to the testing room for over twenty-five minutes before the test. We were on his schedule and apparently our own schedule came second to his. All I wanted was to be treated like a person and recognized. The stress test was supposed to be the conclusive piece of the puzzle to determine if I had a problem with my heart. I wanted and needed the results. I explained several times to the cardiologist that when you have Parkinson's disease it isn't always easy to predict when your medications are going to work. I forewarned him that I couldn't guarantee that I would be able to walk well on a treadmill long enough for an accurate stress test to be done. He insisted that I would do fine.

In less than two and a half minutes on the treadmill my drugs and my legs wore out. To maintain my balance it felt more stabilizing to jog, but the doctor didn't want me to do that. At this point, frustrated Dr. Grandpa got downright irritated and even a little angry with me for not keeping pace with his inclined treadmill.

In a defeatist voice, he yelled, "We're done!"

"I can keep going," I said.

Once again, and in a disappointed manner, he repeated, "We're done!"

I felt fine. I just couldn't keep pace with the treadmill.

I had asked him earlier for the results of my echocardiogram from the previous week and he had told me I could only get those results after the stress test. As if in retaliation for my ending this most sacred of tests early, he coldly blurted out, "Your heart is slightly enlarged and inflamed. There is a buildup of fluid along the wall of the heart cavity. I'll recommend a regimen of beta blockers and ACE inhibitors to your doctor and you can talk with him."

I asked him, "Are there side effects?"

"There are always side effects," he snapped back.

My wife asked him, "What do you call this?"

His answer was, "Cardiomyopathy."

My wife and I were stunned. We didn't know much about this condition, but it sounded horrible.

Our minds were running through all sorts of potential scenarios that might occur if I had to contend with both PD and heart disease. Rather than stand next to me and help me absorb what he'd just told me or help me make decisions, Dr. Grandpa scooted all around the room cleaning countertops and disposing of waste. Dr. Grandpa had delivered his message with the iciest of touches and we were paying the price. Like a blur in the corner of my disbelieving eyes, he slipped out of the exam room and into the hallway without telling us what to do or expect. Our heads were swimming with questions and utter shock. He wasn't about to be kind or compassionate to me or my wife.

The ride home was mostly silent, as Angela and I both attempted to make sense of our experience in the doctor's office. I wasn't going to accept his diagnosis without knowing a great deal more. Why hadn't he told me more or given me more information? Did I need to cut sodium out of my diet? Could I exercise safely? What could I do and not do before I began taking the beta-blocker and ACE inhibitor medications that he was prescribing? What the heck was cardiomyopathy?

The doctor had dropped his bomb on me and my wife just before Christmas. He said he would make drug recommendations to my general practitioner when we were done, and then left us with questions unanswered. He was so matter-of-fact and dismissive that it was scary. I didn't need my hand held by him; I had Angela for that. What I needed was reassurance and information, and he failed miserably in delivering these! I wasn't prepared for the bear trap to snap as abruptly as it had. I'd thought the doctor was on my side. He wasn't.

A week later, as requested by Dr. Grandpa, I went to see my generic practitioner (yes, I do mean generic). My GP gave me the same sweet song and dance as Dr. Grandpa. He said I was to be started on a beta-blocker and ACE inhibitor. It was then I truly questioned my doctor's understanding of my unique condition and my best interest. He was my doctor. He knew I had Parkinson's and that I was taking several medications—and even if he'd forgotten it should have been all over my file, which possibly he hadn't read.

I have low blood pressure and my current meds keep it around 100–110 over 70 or 80. That's low. If I took these new heart drugs they were going to lower my blood pressure further. The last thing I needed was new additions to the drug soup I was taking, especially ones that would exacerbate my fatigue, dizziness, lightheadedness, sleepiness, and who knew what else.

I told my GP flat out, "This doesn't feel right. I want to see another cardiologist and get a second opinion."

His response? "Fine, but in the meantime you should start the new drugs."

I told him I would think about it. Then I went home and called the records department to request a complete copy of my file. I didn't tell the office, but I was done with my GP. If you know your body and your doctor isn't listening to you, you have to take a walk. That voice of reason in my brain was yelling at me that I needed to go get more information. The information that I should have received from my cardiologist would have to come to me from somewhere else.

I called my friends who are doctors and searched the Web. According to the sources I consulted, my heart was dying and there wasn't much I could do about it. Some said to lower my sodium and liquid intake. Some said exercise could help, and others said to be cautious about exercising. Some said only a heart transplant could save me.

It was clear that I needed another professional to examine me. Next stop, get a second opinion. This time I wanted to be wiser about whom I spoke with. I called my neurologist to get a recommendation from her for both a general practitioner and a cardiologist with a better understanding of PD who would give me a second opinion. She gave me a name of a cardiologist and I called for an appointment with Dr. Cardio.

Dr. Cardio was a high energy woman who was slightly nervous, highly intelligent, and an efficient listener. She seemed to me like an oasis in a desert of medical incompetence. All of her nurses, technicians, and even she took notes and kept their records on electronic tablets rather than on scribbling pieces of paper that would have to be transcribed.

After reviewing the information, reviewing my heart, listening to me, and hearing why I had such limited faith in my former GP and Dr. Grandpa, Dr. Cardio felt it was best to start from scratch. I told her of the frustration with my meds wearing out during the stress test. She asked, "Why didn't you do a chemical stress test?" Well, I had never heard of a chemical stress test. She explained that chemical stress tests are close to 90 percent accurate, whereas treadmill stress tests have only 50 percent accuracy. I didn't have to get on a treadmill?! This was news to me!

Why hadn't Dr. Grandpa thought of that?

Before the chemical stress test, Dr. Cardio performed another echocardiogram. It came back normal. The next week, I had the chemical stress test and it also proved normal. Dr. Cardio and I were perplexed. What did the other doctors see that she hadn't?

Maybe I had an intermittent problem like when your car makes a knocking or dinging sound only for you, but refuses to do it for your mechanic at the garage. To test this theory, Dr. Cardio suggested I wear a "halter" for a day. While I wasn't sure how wearing women's clothing was going to help, she explained that the halter would record my heart continuously for twenty-four hours. We did that and it, too, proved that my heart was working just fine.

Here is what I found out after my second opinion: Some Parkinson's disease medications can cause palpitations and extra heartbeats. It took two doctors to uncover this fact for me. Had I not gone for a second opinion, I could be taking unnecessary meds with unwanted side effects and severe consequences. It amazes and perplexes me, but had I not gotten this second look at my condition, I could have done massive harm to myself—perhaps even died.

The lesson is: No one knows you and your body better than you. If you don't know it well, then it's time to get in touch now. Self-awareness is a crucial component to self-healing. I am not a doctor, but consider this: If any of your doctors ask you to make a radical change in your health regimen and you have any doubts at all about the potential consequences of the change, then you need a second opinion to ease your mind and avoid possible mistakes.

I never received an acknowledgement, an apology, an email, or even a Christmas card from the general practitioner or the first cardiologist. Neither of them cared about me either as a patient or as a person. About two years later, my general practitioner left his group to go out on his own. He called me to invite me to become a patient in his new office. I asked him if he would come to a Reiki class that I was teaching. He told me he wouldn't come.

I told him the same thing.

CHAPTER 7
Doctors Are Human

Learn from others and instill knowledge where you can.

Some lessons come from the most unusual situations. Throughout most of my cardiology visits, I had remained pretty stable and showed few Parkinson's symptoms. The doctor was aware that I had PD and understood what it meant, or so I thought. At my last visit, however, she walked into the office and her face went pale at the sight of me. It was early morning and my meds were working a little too well. I had begun having dyskinesia and was finding it a challenge to stay seated in the padded office furniture.

"We're going to have to reschedule this appointment," she told us. I was making her nervous.

"Wait. Just give me a minute," I pled. The stress and tension in the room escalated. I knew that if I couldn't gather myself together immediately she was going to walk out and I was going to have to come back again. It wasn't like I was doing my uncontrollable undulating dance on command. With the help of my wife, Angela, and meditation I was able to qualm the excess energy of the dyskinesia. As I calmed down, the tension in the room dissipated.

My doctor felt compelled to share the fact that she experiences anxiety. At first I was concerned that she wouldn't be a good doctor because she doesn't deal well with pressure, but then I realized the error of my thinking. I realized that she is a professional and human, too. She had been efficient, a good listener, and helped me stay off beta-blockers and ACE inhibitors. She is a good doctor and she treated me well. We all have our issues, illnesses, and our weaknesses.

By remaining vigilant in my care, I have been fortunate to keep a good working relationship with my doctors. I am able to maintain overall good health by keeping regular appointments with my dentist (twice a year), dermatologist (once a year or more), and neurologist (every four to six months), and by visiting my internist (for my yearly checkup or as needed). This is not to say that you may want to see your doctor more often than me.

I have had several neurologists over the past twenty years. I am grateful that I have maintained a relationship of mutual respect with my current neurologist, Dr. Linda Sigmund. She is one of the best and most respected neurologists and movement disorder specialists in the United States. I will admit that, at times, our egos collided and we came very close to parting ways because we were not communicating well.

If a doctor only sees you for fifteen to twenty minutes every few months, only a meager slice of your life is revealed. As both Dr. Sigmund and I are active within the Parkinson's community, however, we both see each other outside the examination room. Slowly, I think she began to see my improvement in and out of her office. Prior to our understanding, she had suggested the option of deep brain stimulation (DBS), which surprised me, because my condition had not deteriorated to that level and my symptoms did not seem to fit the criteria that DBS is meant to assist. All I can guess is that an occasional bout of stress induced dyskinesia, which DBS may or may not help resolve, was her reasoning for the mention. Since that talk, we concluded that my complementary therapies were having a major benefit to my symptoms and DBS wasn't necessary. I was seeing change, and now so was my neurologist.

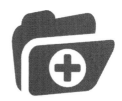

CHAPTER 8
Keep Good Records and Remind Your Doctors

Vigilance and good record keeping is very important with a chronic illness.

There is a fundamental breakdown in medicine when it comes to doctors and their patients who are dealing with chronic illnesses. As if we don't have enough to focus on, it is also our job to see that our myriad of tests and reports are seen and shared by our full cadre of doctors. It is our job to remind them of our drug regimen and what exactly is on the laundry list of drugs that we take. If we don't look out for ourselves, accidents, mistakes, and oversights may occur.

You are your best advocate. To expect a doctor who sees you for only ten to fifteen minutes at intervals of between two and six months to know the nuances of your condition as well as you do is unrealistic. Unless your various doctors share information and are willing to do an in-depth exploration of your case, without you watching closely to make sure they are looking at the right facts—and the complete facts—some important facts may fall through the cracks.

Here are a few simple guidelines you may find useful:

- Keep good records of your medications. If one doctor adds a new drug to your regimen, be in charge of notifying the other doctors you see, so they can update their files.
- Track your responses to your treatment. Make note of any symptoms or changes in your condition that you experience. Your doctor may be of help to you to distinguish between side effects of taking meds and signs of the progression of Parkinson's.
- Read the package inserts that come with your medications and make note of possible side effects. Talk with your pharmacist if you have questions.
- Read about drugs, treatments, and tests on reputable medical and patient advocacy sites on the Internet; however, *be cautious about believing everything you read*. Information found online has not necessarily been reviewed and could be wildly inaccurate. Read with an eye toward knowing what kinds of questions to ask your doctor and to be informed of possible alarm signals.

- Have your pharmacist check the database for possible adverse drug interactions.
- Create a portable binder of your medical history, which includes contact names, phone numbers, emails, and street addresses of every doctor and institution that has treated or tested you, as well as your up-to-date insurance information.
- Take notes or use a voice recorder at your appointment.
- When you have a new test done and receive results, be sure to send a copy to each of your doctors for whom this is appropriate (examples, neurologist, general practitioner, internist, and cardiologist), and so on.

Ask Your Doctor for a "Health and Travel Document"
It's a good idea to get a letter from your physician and/or neurologist describing and verifying your physical condition. You may want to draft this letter and have it typed up on your doctor's professional letterhead. Be sure it is officially signed by your doctor. Modify the wording of your letter to fit your needs and personal concerns, including mentioning the type of disease and symptoms you often experience, or medication side effects, and the different needs you may have for managing your particular condition.

Once you have the letter in hand, scan the document and save it. Make several copies of the original document and file copies in a safe place. Put a copy in a filing cabinet and laminate the original that is on letterhead. Almost any FedEx Office or other copy shop can laminate and scan documents for you. Keep a portable copy tucked inside your wallet. Your doctor may ask for a small fee to write and print a letter but it is worth it.

You'll find a safety letter valuable to you when you travel through airport security stations, or have trouble getting necessary words out when speaking with authorities, flight attendants, and first responders. You'll find this letter of benefit when travelling and working with airport personnel, Transportation Security Officers, police, or anyone who needs a quick assessment of your condition.

Here's an example of how it could read:

RE: John Doe, Patient #1234

To Whom It May Concern:

Mr. John Doe, the bearer of this letter, is my patient and under my care and treatment. He is afflicted with early onset of Parkinson's disease. This illness may cause him to move awkwardly or erratically. Unless Mr. Doe tells you otherwise, there should be no reason for concern about his movement. The medications that he is taking can cause uncontrollable flailing or shaking, but it will wear off.

Parkinson's patients can display numerous symptoms such as: balance issues, gait problems, stumbling, and uncontrollable running to maintain balance, slurred or stuttered speech, stiffness, tremor, falling, and hunched posture. At times, please be aware that Mr. Doe is susceptible to these symptoms and actions.

Mr. Doe's condition is not a threat to anyone. Please be patient, understanding, and considerate. Parkinson's patients show more symptoms when rushed, stressed, and put under pressure. Thank you.

Sincerely,

[Signature]

Doctor's Name, M.D.

CHAPTER 9
How to Talk
to Doctors

We are observed, but unseen.
We are heard, but not listened to.
Our health is impaired, but our spirits are intact.
Overlooked and underestimated,
Often ignored and frequently misunderstood,
Illness finds us and wellness takes a vacation.
Hidden in plain sight are we.

Speaking with a doctor can be like talking to a foreigner whose language you've never heard before. You won't necessarily understand the doctor and the doctor won't necessarily understand you. Miscommunication can be aggravating, frustrating, emotionally draining, and confusing.

Here are some suggestions for an easier and more productive visit to your doctor's office.
- Be prepared and on time for your appointments.
- If you believe you will really need extra time,

book two appointment slots in a row. And, if you ultimately discover your doctor is routinely unwilling or incapable of giving you the time that you need, you may want to consider going elsewhere to meet your medical needs.

- Bring a spouse or care partner, a daughter, a son, a parent, or a close friend to your appointment to ask the questions or bring up the concerns that you forget to address with your doctor. Having someone with you is good support and your companion may take notes for you so you can pay attention to the doctor. You may want to record the appointment with a voice recorder.

- Educate yourself as best you can on your illness beforehand. By researching and learning about what is happening to your body, you empower yourself and make the doctor's job easier. Use the Internet, libraries, newsletters, blogs, and support groups to stay in touch and be informed in research, trials, and new therapies in your illness. There is so much happening in the field of neurological medicine, which is advancing quickly, that your doctor may miss a breakthrough here and there. Most doctors respect a knowledgeable patient and appreciate a patient who understands his or her disease and medicines. By taking a primary role in educating yourself on your condition, both you and your doctor are able to communicate about your condition.

- Bring your medical journal or binder with you, and be sure it holds the latest updates.

- To make the most of your appointment,

come in with a list of changes or concerns for discussion. Prepare a list of questions, side effects, or anything new that you are experiencing. Be ready to share news of symptoms, no matter how small, with your doctor.

- Remember that doctors are busy and have only a short time to talk with you. Because they are on a strict schedule, you get better results from coming in prepared. Just make sure to address the highest priority items on your "to discuss" list, first.

- Sadly, medical practices sometimes get so big that patients get lost in the shuffle. If you and your doctor have something in common (for example, you went to the same school, share a love of dogs, you both shoot nature photography, you go to the same church) let the doctor know. If your doctor feels a common bond with you, your doctor is more likely to identify with you on a human level and remember you when you come in.

- Ask questions about your treatment to show that you care. Proving to your doctor that you care as much as you do about the status of your health naturally reinforces your commitment to your health and it also makes your doctor's job easier.

- Take thorough notes during the appointment. With the permission of everybody in the room you might choose to record the conversation. Most smart phones can record audio, or you can put an app on them that does.

- Be personable, but professional, in conduct. Be respectful and yet don't take everything your doctor says as the complete, one and only truth.

DON'T LABEL ME OR MY ILLNESS

Don't allow yourself to be bullied into a particular solution. If you have questions or concerns about a medication or treatment that your doctor wants to prescribe, then you are entitled to ask about risks, side effects, benefits, and any other potential concerns that you may have. After all, it's your body. You also have to live with the consequences of decisions that are made. Feel free to ask for a second opinion if you just cannot gain resolution about what's being advised.

It is ingrained in our western culture not to question the authority of doctors. There is no doubt that doctors provide vital and life-saving services, but there are times, such as when you are dealing with life-or-death situations, that you have the right to question your doctor. If you rely solely on a doctor's advice for treatment, you may well cheat yourself out of an opportunity to improve your condition. Although they don't advertise it much, scientists and doctors don't yet fully understand the complexity of the human body and brain. It is their lack of complete understanding that I believe repeals the doctor's right to act as if they are looking into a crystal ball and predicting a patient's future outcome.

You must do your part to get better. Feeling better begins with making the mental shift to know and believe that you can get better. The medical community in general believes that people with Parkinson's, like people with many other illnesses, only get worse—period. They therefore provide us with little hope for improving our condition and when speaking to us often use terms like: "chronic" and "degenerative." It is rare that I meet a doctor who prescribes hope and positive thinking to his or her patients.

Positive thinking and hope can help people get through the most traumatic of events. Feats of superhuman strength in times of crisis, heroism under severe pressure, survival under extreme conditions, and the ability to push the body beyond its breaking point are just some of the unexplained medical phenomenon that science can't fully dissect. Why shouldn't everyone be capable of such feats?

Programming us to accept that we will only get worse and feel worse can be as dangerous as it is powerful. This is the *nocebo* effect (a negative placebo). When a patient is diagnosed with an illness and the doctor tells a patient that there is "no hope," the negative reinforcement can have devastating consequences on the patient's whole being. Without being false or betraying a professional oath, the same doctor could say, "We have no medical answer for your illness at this time, so I suggest you investigate other potential therapies that may benefit you that western culture has yet to embrace, but which show great (or even some) promise."

Of course, you probably won't hear this type of advice from most medical doctors. Yet shifting the standard outlook from grim to hopeful could revolutionize medicine and improve the lives of the ill seeking a cure or just a better life. There is power in keeping positive.

A Challenge to Doctors

• Refrain from treating me like a number.

• Be my partner or teammate in my recovery and treatment.

• Remember my name.

• Don't be so quick to rush to surgery when other choices are available.

• There is a place for creativity in medicine. Think a little differently on my behalf.

• Understand that I need handholding some-times as much as I need physical relief.

• Don't take me at face value. I have a life and a personality outside of your office.

• Really observe me and listen to what I say.

• Ask questions and hear the answers.

• Treat me as an equal.

• Accept that my care partner or family member has valuable information to offer you that may be pertinent to my condition.

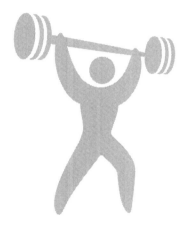

PART TWO

Living with Parkinson's Disease

CHAPTER 10
Coping with a Diagnosis

"It all depends on how we look at things, and not on how they are in themselves."—Carl Jung

Receiving a diagnosis of Parkinson's disease will make you stop and consider your future. It's a sobering reality to have to get a grip on. Frankly, now is a good time to evaluate what it is you want to accomplish during the remaining years of your life. The questions to ask are important and probably obvious. Here are a few that I found most helpful to me:

- How am I going to continue to work?
- Do I tell my employer?
- What do I do now?
- How do I tell my spouse, child, relative, or friend?
- Do I begin medicines or wait?
- Do I need a neurologist even if I have a fine

primary physician?
- If Parkinson's is chronic and progressive, is there anything I can do about it?
- Where can I go for emotional support and information on living with PD?

These are just some of the many questions that arise when someone is newly diagnosed.

It is important to know that there are resources and loads of valuable organizations that can help you answer your questions. There is an amazing network of Parkinson's patients across the United States and around the world. Many of us have been where you've been. While PD can be, and often is, a very individualized illness, sharing stories and information proves that many of us are facing a common situation. It is vital to understand that you are not alone with this illness and there is much that you can do to live well, on a daily basis.

I hope that the information and resources in this book answer your questions or lead you to resources that will.

CHAPTER 11
Parkinson's Doesn't Mean the End

When the road ahead is dark and steep, push on.
When your body says, "Enough," but your mind says, "Go," push on.
When your goal is true of purpose and ever so near, push on.
When life gets hard, seek the solution and push on

Look at Parkinson's disease as a challenge. It is an obstacle, a hurdle you can overcome by delving deeply inside to discover who you are. Everyone has flaws in body, mind, or character, and disease may help us to address these imperfections. With time and effort, this can become your opportunity to learn from the humility that comes with disease. If you look deeply in your being, you will find grace and compassion there. Disease makes for a powerful teacher.

I make no claims to be any more "enlightened" or smarter than any others, whether they are dealing with an illness or are symptom free. As you go through fear, anger, sadness, loss, and acceptance of your illness, realize that this experience you're having is about more than just you. Illness has an impact on you and on all those who care about you.

For myself, I decided to use my illness as an opportunity to teach, change, and inspire the world with my story. Among other things, my intention is always to help doctors and other members of the medical community understand and serve their Parkinsonian patients better.

FINDING MEANING IN DISEASE

When disease strikes, it is usually shockingly unexpected. News of a Parkinson's diagnosis is a jolt that we are unwilling to accept or comprehend. Few of us would have expected illness to invade our bodies and interfere with our way of life. This happens to other people. None of us wants chronic illness, but perhaps, if we remain both cognizant and insightful, we can discover life lessons in it that could only have come from enduring the hardships of illness. Disease provides us with a chance for self-discovery that may not always be obvious.

Keep your wits about you and maintain perspective as you move forward. Hope is a vital element in preparing your body for its battle to maintain health. You must focus your mind on getting well. Visualization and meditation are powerful tools that you may want to explore. Use any tools you can find to lift your spirits, focus on wellness, and manage frustrations.

One of the greatest perspectives to embrace is that change is a reality of life. Like the changes that accompany aging, personal growth, and receiving an education, the changes related to illness teach us an appreciation for the "now." Illness reminds us that life is to be appreciated in the present moment. There never is another time available to us.

Illness wakes us up to what is of true importance. It is the instrument that life taps us on the shoulder with to remind us of our impermanence on this planet. Life is about appreciating those we care about while we can. Illness can bring out the very best of our nature and perspective. It reminds us of our humanity and our vulnerability.

MISSION: LIVING WITH ILLNESS

Love your life for what you can make of it. The hard times in our lives are tests of our ingenuity, strength, tenacity, and courage. Look inward and find the piece of yourself that refuses to give up. Your mission has begun and now is the time to make the most of it.

We were all given some sort of baggage that we must deal with, mend, forget, and discard. Each of us is constricted in some way. We build our own personal prisons in our minds. Whether we build that prison ourselves or it is dealt to us by the hand of fate, we must first learn that as much as we humans love to be in control, rarely are we the masters of our own destiny. The evening news is full of reports of floods, earthquakes, and hurricanes that remind us that while we might be able to alter our existence to some degree, we can't control Mother Nature. And such is also the case with PD and most other diseases: We can't control them, but we may be able to work with a disease or overcome it.

In the occurrence of Parkinson's disease, the body becomes uncontrollable. While medication and medical breakthroughs show great promise, we are still facing a daily war with our own bodies. Thanks to new medications, PD patients receive some of the necessary ammunition to win some of the battles—at least for a while. While we may be victims of a disease that limits our bodies, PD has the capability of enhancing our senses. PD patients are sensitive beings with a heightened awareness and caring for those around us. Our illness often gives us a perspective on life that a healthy person may take for granted.

We are not at fault for having Parkinson's disease. There is a limited explanation for our neurological differences, but there is no reason for us to try and make sense of our condition other than to accept it. There is a peace that comes with acceptance. While we don't have to give up, we must accept our state and move forward.

Parkinson's disease is a cruel and awkward disease. Unlike diseases that rob the afflicted with debilitating symptoms quickly, Parkinson's pickpockets you over time. Stealthily and silently you may lose various speech, motor, and cognitive functions. You are left never knowing if today will be as good as yesterday. Simple pleasures are what your body is inevitably left to enjoy. By then you can only remember fondly what most people take for granted: activities like skiing, driving, running, dancing, walking, and even dressing yourself. It doesn't have to be this way.

Although we don't like admitting to it, limitations come with PD. We have to learn to compensate for these changes. Most of my life, I have been an avid skier, but as I see my balance deteriorate and discover that I am having more difficulty walking, I am accepting the fact that skiing may no longer be a sport that fits my ability. My days of skiing may be over for now, but with time and searching, I may find another sport. I gave up tennis for years and started playing again. I was overjoyed to be back on the court. My point is that just because PD has taken something that I enjoy doesn't mean that my life is over. It is up to us to fill the voids in our lives.

Focus on whatever makes you happy. As your body changes and your symptoms evolve, what once pleased you may not be as enjoyable as it used to be. Be it a loss in taste, difficulty with vision, or some unexpected side effect, you must find a replacement for the enjoyment that has been taken from you. If you can no longer ski, take up photography. You must learn to compensate and compromise. Don't stop seeking new options.

Your mind and body may be out of sync, but with work I believe one can overcome many of the symptoms that come with PD. You can find the strength you need to go on in yourself, from support groups, from friends and family, or from inspirational writing, music, film, or your faith. Parkinson's is not the end. You have a choice.

CHAPTER 12
This Disease Isn't Fair

"Hope sees the invisible, feels the intangible, and achieves the impossible."—Anonymous

Living with PD is a daily challenge. From one moment to the next, it is a game of chance. As durable and complicated as the human body may be, it is also fragile. In PD, unless medication, diet, circulation, and all other related neurological factors coincide and work in harmony, the Parkinsonian will face some sort of wrath from the body. Like any complicated instrument, if these factors don't coalesce he or she may face a range of symptoms from limited motion to excessive motion. Parkinsonians must make the most of the days when the body's functions are orchestrated, and weather the days of dysfunction as best as humanly possible.

I often think of the statement: "No one ever

said life was fair." The word "fair" is a deceptive word with an elusive meaning. Fair is a concept, not a reality. Everyone has a different perspective of what is fair. Fairness is a degree or a label, like "pretty" or "nice." Without interpretation, it means little. What is fair to one person may seem completely unjust to another.

No one is immune from pain, nor is anyone void of pleasure. Cold hard reality can hurt, but to our benefit it also can open our eyes to what is, not just what could be. Too often we live for the future and not for the present. It is easy to lose that mindful, centered state and run out of hope or to escape our daily reality. Remain focused on helping yourself!

There can be a loneliness that accompanies PD. Loneliness is a universal reaction that afflicts all of us at some point in our lives. If you feel lonely, don't let the illness beat you down. Your emotional well-being may change like the weather. You owe it to yourself to hang in during the lows and do your best to maintain a positive outlook, knowing that the "sun will shine again." Cut yourself some slack for feeling the way you feel.

That said, you will achieve very little with a negative attitude. At best, all you'll do with a negative attitude is alienate those around you. You have a chance to make a change in yourself and those around you for the better. Parkinson's has entered your life—accept the challenge.

Bitterness can fester and can eat at you from the inside out. If the mind truly does control and feed the body, then it only makes sense that poisonous thoughts and acrid feelings are unhealthy.

It is my belief, as well as the belief of many others, that we each contribute to our own decline. Whether or not we know it, we make much of our destiny from within ourselves. I believe that we have the capability of change and can adapt as does a chameleon in the wild.

Only through being open in thought and by releasing your mind and heart will you see change in your outlook. The past is the past. Move forward with the wide eyes of the educated student of life. Accept that you sail the ship of your destiny and it's your job to see it safely to port.

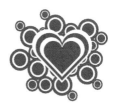

CHAPTER 13
Dealing with Depression

"There are two ways to live: you can live as if nothing is a miracle; you can live as if everything is a miracle."—Albert Einstein

As a generally upbeat person, I wasn't prepared for the lows that can accompany Parkinson's. Depression used to be something that I had only read about; now it's something that I have to deal with periodically. Luckily, I only see depression crop up a few days each year.

Depression can be dangerous and debilitating—if you let it be. You may experience thoughts that no one cares what you're feeling or understands what you're feeling. The feelings that flood you along with such thoughts can be very painful. Even those who don't have illness can feel this way. This painful and negative thought pattern attacks almost everyone at some point. We all have problems and we don't have to be depressed by them. You can beat it.

Remember this: It's not your fault that you got PD. There is no shame in it, just as there's no weakness in expressing emotions, only weakness in avoiding emotions. You can control your thoughts and your emotions, but you'll have to work on your control every day.

Here are nine helpful hints that I use for chasing away the blues.

- If "music has charms to soothe the savage breast," as playwright William Congreve wrote, it should do you some good for your depression. Put on your favorite album, tape, disc, or radio station. If you sing or play an instrument, sing or play along.
- Exercise. Studies have proven that exercise can relieve depression and helps the symptoms of PD.
- Watch a favorite movie or a good comedy. Whether it's slapstick or standup, if it makes you smile, then it has done its job. If it makes you laugh, even better.
- Sit down and list ten things you are thankful for.
- Surround yourself with inspirational photos. It's easy to take the little things for granted, whether it's the food we eat, the people we know, or the sunrise. Seeing images reminds us of what we are grateful for, and helps us to remember on a daily basis.
- Call a friend.
- Get a pet. Go out to your local animal shelter and bring home a furry friend. You'll be saving a life while you're enriching your own. Animals

love unconditionally and many need a loving home.

- Do your best to keep a positive attitude in everything you do. Although this may seem much easier said than done, if you monitor what you are thinking (as compared to what you are feeling), you'll be halfway there on the road to beating the blues.
- Try writing a poem, a song, or a short story. You'll find that expressing your feelings on paper can be a wonderful release of tension. Writing can be cathartic.

If your depression feels too severe to deal with by yourself, get professional help from a counselor and call your doctor. Only a trained medical professional should treat severe depression. Monitor your moods and mood swings.

CHAPTER 14
Be Good to Yourself

"Make the best use of what is in your power, and take the rest as it happens."—Epictetus

Parkinson's disease may change your life, but it doesn't have to ruin it. You owe it to yourself to find pleasure wherever you can and to be as good to yourself as you can—as long as you can do so and remain within the boundaries of your financial means, of course. Whether by giving yourself the gift of an occasional night out, a massage, or a vacation, be kind to yourself.

For many who get ill, either with Parkinson's or another disease, one of the biggest traps is forgetting to have fun. Something as simple as hearing live music in a club, watching a funny film, engaging in an interesting conversation, reading a thrilling novel, or playing an action-packed video game can be a wonderful release of tension and a pleasurable way to overcome the blues.

A favorite food or a decadent dessert that you rarely indulge in can be a wonderful thing for you to look forward to, and enjoy. Plan ahead. Whether it is a brief overnight getaway, a concert in the park, seeing friends, or watching the latest critically acclaimed film, plan to do something that you want to do, regularly. It doesn't hurt to keep an actual list of what you want to do.

It is important to stay realistic about your abilities and resources. Avoid setting yourself up for disappointment by overreaching in your expectations. Don't plan an around-the-world escapade if you can't afford it or if you don't have the stamina to endure such an adventure. Adhere to and accept your limitations, but also get out in the world and live your life!

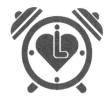

CHAPTER 15
Timing in Parkinson's Disease May Be Everything

Timing medication takes diligence, practice, and a dash of luck.

D o you find yourself losing track of time? Do you ever miss a dose of your medicine because you get distracted from the task at hand? Well, you are not alone. This is a common problem for Parkies, as we somehow find keeping track of time to be a challenge. Multitasking is a mistake for someone with this illness. If an orderly and well-defined task list is created, stating a specific time of completion, there is a much better chance for a given task to be fulfilled.

So much of being capable revolves around

scheduling your medicines according to the events of your day. Keeping up on a simple daily regimen can feel like a full-time job in itself, and the longer you have this illness the more you'll recognize the importance of being diligent in monitoring how your body is reacting to your medicines. Too little medicine in your system and signs of PD show through. Too much medicine in your system unleashes side effects. When your day is not going to be a routine day, however, you also have to plan for your activities.

On top of maximizing your medicines, being capable is related to variables such as how well you slept the night before, how much stress you are under, what you ate—and how much—and even your mood and state of mind. Even the weather can play a part in how well you function on a given day. Although I have no empirical research to back the next statement up, I know it's been true for me: Weather has an impact on my condition and whether or not my meds work well that day.

Here are five suggestions for getting more out of your medicines and every day.

- Wearing a watch that beeps on the hour can keep you aware of the time of day and alert you to when you may be due for your next dose of medication. There are some elaborate and helpful timers and pill box systems for sale to keep you on track. If you are interested in these, just Google "electronic pill box" or "pill timers." For your smart phone or tablet, there are also apps on dosages and timing. (See the Resources section.)
- I find that ingesting a little caffeine (in the

form of coffee or tea) along with my medication speeds the uptake. This may not work
for everyone, and if you have heart problems
or a problem with caffeine, don't try it and
talk to your doctor.

- Calm your mind and body for at least five
minutes a day with a meditation. As you get
more used to the experience of meditation,
you can do it for longer periods if you like.
Try different types and see which ones work
best for you. A local yoga studio should be a
good resource.

- Keep as physically fit and active as you can.
Build an exercise regimen that you can stick
to, and try to incorporate stretching, balance,
walking, and maybe some weight training
into the mix. Consult with your doctor and
a qualified physical therapist or trainer who
understands PD to design the right workout
routine for you.

- Challenge your mind daily. Doing a daily
crossword or Sudoku puzzle is a wonderful
way to get your brain going for the day.

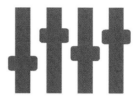

CHAPTER 16
Structure Your Life to Gain Some Control

"Look to this day, for it is life. In its brief course, with all the realities and truths of existence, the joy of growth, the glory of action, the splendor of beauty...today well lived makes every yester-day a memory of happiness and every tomorrow a vision of hope. Look well, therefore, to this day."
—Sanskrit proverb

Personally, I believe in seeking out any poten-tially life-improving therapy and/or proce-dure as long as it isn't harmful, costly, painful or damaging. I try never to allow my PD symptoms to interfere with my quality of life or my respon-sibilities, work, movement, and social obligations. That being said, I also have to weigh my symptoms against my objectives every single day to see which ones will take precedence over the others.

How you structure or re-structure your life to fit the disease is a balancing act. It's a way of coping by accommodating your symptoms, meds, stress, diet, need for sleep, and other outside intangibles that may impact you. With Parkinson's disease, as with any neurological disorder, schedules and daily agendas are most beneficial when they're followed with consistency. Creating order and establishing a daily regimen is comforting for you and your care partners. Managing the many variables in your life reduces undue stress and helps you remain calm.

When stricken with illness of any kind, people may feel a tremendous loss of control. Whether it is a loss of say over the protocols of their treatment, loss of body function, or loss of speech, people rarely, if ever, are given the luxury of steering their own "ship", entirely. However, they are ultimately in control of making critical decisions that will alter their long-term health.

"Control" is a funny word when you use it in the same sentence as Parkinson's disease, for several reasons. After having met thousands of PD patients, I can say that unscientifically, they are often intelligent, motivated, overachievers, who want to be in control of their own fates. In her book, *You Can Heal Your Life* (Hay House, 1999), Louise Hay even refers to PD's cause as "fear and an intense desire to control everything and everyone."

Speaking from experience, I readily admit that when I choose to release my desire to try to manipulate things, events, and people that are out of my control, I feel better. Over the course of my life, I have come to realize that there is a natural progression for us all to find the balance of our own affairs. I can be a resource to those people in my life without putting demands on them or forcing unwarranted judgments that are often unfair and completely unnecessary. If I control anything, rather than trying to control people's actions and things that have nothing to do with me, it should be improving who I am, how I feel, and how I treat those around me. With most any disease, can come a sense and fear of loss. When dealing with the unknown, it is frightening, and that's what happens in any medical crisis. There is nothing easy about dealing with disease. It will change some elements of your life regardless of what you want. Control is a squishy ball of goo that only you can manipulate. Control is an illusion that we build for ourselves.

Relinquish control of the parts of your life that you logically know you cannot change. Whether it's the weather or the stock market, accept that life is just as it is and that you are how you are, for the moment. Take a deep breath. Let the stress just melt away.

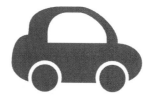

CHAPTER 17
Driving

Excuses can't change fact.

If there is one crucial question that both young-on-set and older Parkinsonians face, it's, "When do I give up the keys and leave the driving to someone else?" At age thirty, I made the decision to stop driving and it was terribly difficult. I had come to the realization that my reactions were slowing. My reflexes just weren't fast enough for the Beltway around Washington, D.C. More importantly, I knew that I could not in good conscience endanger innocent motorists, my family, myself, or cyclists, pedestrians, and free-roving animals just because I was selfishly unwilling to relinquish my automobile. I changed to accommodate the fact that my body had changed. My driving ability had diminished, so it was only natural that for the safety and security of my community and my own self-preservation that I leave the driving in our household to my wife.

I have driven with numerous Annie Hall-like drivers with Parkinson's disease (remember the scenes in the movie from the trip to Long Island?), who have a total disregard and lack of awareness for fellow drivers and a carefree interpretation of the rules of the road. I have seen them miss stop signs and perform U-turns where signs explicitly say that it is unlawful.

Let's face it. Giving up driving doesn't have to be your loss of freedom—even though it may take some readjustment of your life and a shift in how you perceive real freedom. If you get a little creative and find some flexibility in your approach, you can make a smooth transition.

Here are some questions that you may consider in advance of this decision:

- When you drive, are you a threat to others, your family, or yourself?
- Is your reaction time sufficiently fast either to brake or to accelerate fast enough to avoid a potential accident?
- Have you had a fender bender or worse in the last few months? Any close calls?
- Is mass transit an option for getting around in the area where you live?
- Could you share a ride or get a ride from friends, family, or spouse?
- Are there other transportation options that your city or state may provide?
- Have you talked with national and local Parkinson's organizations about people in your area that may be able to assist you?
- Have you researched ride share programs

and city or state programs in your area?

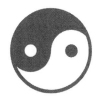

CHAPTER 18
Two-headed Monster

My disease chose me. There must be a reason.
I know not why my brain declared treason.
A traitor to my body and my muscle control,
Parkinson's disease can take quite a toll.

I did not choose it, but it is a great teacher.
It's a two-headed monster that's not a pretty creature.

One head teaches patience and slows the pace of life.
The other causes problems and creates a lot of strife.

The key is how you deal with life and all it throws at you.
Either step up for the challenge or watch it pass on

through.

Your character and attitude will see you through the
fight.
Do what you can to battle this disease and keep the
enemy in sight.

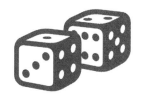

CHAPTER 19
Sickness
Happens

"Courage is being scared to death and saddling up anyway."—John Wayne

It seems so easy for our government to send men and women off to war to die, and often soldiers are forgotten once they're injured or get ill. As a society, we hide our ill or choose to look away. We sweep dust under the rug and pour dioxin in the river in the dead of night. We pump toxins into our air, food, and water and then wonder, with bewilderment, why we're getting ill. We have a healthcare system that doesn't pay to maintain our health, but pays us after the fact.

Illness may strike at any time. For me, that time came at the age of seventeen. I was fortunate that my tremors were mild and rare at first. Back then, in my adolescence, tremors only came out under stressful conditions. Along with the tremors, I noticed a change in my posture. The soles of my shoes were being worn unevenly from my shuffling and the way I was dragging my feet. The point is this: health is tenuous and can change overnight even for young people. You need to know that how well you cope with your illness at the start can mark how those close to you perceive you from then on. Your attitude is what will make the difference in how others treat you. No one wants to hear constant complaining about your condition or what isn't working.

Fortunately, Parkinson's can bring out the best in people. In my experience, we Parkinsonians can be a beacon of hope and inspiration to others. Illness highlights what is important in our lives and clarifies our personal mission. At this time, medical experts have no cure for PD. As strange as it may sound, I don't know that if there were a cure for PD that I'd take it. Why? Because PD heightens our sensitivity to those around us, it heightens our awareness of our feelings, and it heightens our understanding of what it is like to be different, which means we are able to be empathetic and compassionate to a diversity of people in different circumstances.

No one is immune from illness. Whether you suffer from chronic fatigue; nagging, full-blown, throbbing migraines; some form of cancer; or Parkinson's disease. You probably never planned for illness to play a role in your daily life. Just getting through life some days is hard enough let alone getting through a day fighting a daily battle with a chronic illness.

The reality of our disease stinks, but we are

lucky thanks to the present advances in medicine. We must maintain some perspective on our disease and on life. We are fortunate for current drugs (and those forthcoming), which have helped so many of us. At the same time, we must also create peace within ourselves, because this is a healthier way to live. Medicines and doctors can only do so much. The more we take responsibility for trying to improve ourselves and maintain or even reverse our condition, the better off we will be.

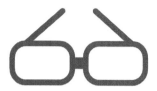

CHAPTER 20
Ten Tips for Dealing with Parkinson's Disease

"The clock is running. Make the most of today. Time waits for no man. Yesterday is history. Tomorrow is a mystery. Today is a gift. That's why it is called the present." —Alice Morse Earle

Here are ten tips for dealing with PD.

- Look deep inside yourself and face your disease head on. Understanding its symptoms and possible treatments for it would be a good start.
- Seek inspiration around you. There is courage, strength, and beauty all around us in children, animals, nature, scenery, books, music, film, art, and spirit.

- Identify a hero or role model; be inspired by someone you look up to. Get invigorated by someone who overcame adversity. This will strengthen your survival instinct. People are doing amazing feats and overcoming huge obstacles. You can, too!
- Build a network of family and friends. Create a community of people that energizes you. Find or develop a support group, or at least participate in an online chat room for people with Parkinson's or your specific illness.
- Get involved in efforts to fund research, awareness, and attend lectures and symposiums for your disease. Your actions can lead to change. Share your story.
- Consider going vegetarian. I have loved animals all my life. It just felt right to go vegetarian. After being vegetarian for over twenty years, I can say I feel clearer in my head, my medication works better and my digestion is better.
- Continue to dream and don't lose hope. What inspires you? Pursue it!
- Be open and willing to explore new treatment options that may offer relief, but which are not invasive and cannot harm you.
- Take charge of your life and body. Exercise as best you can.
- Do what you can when you can, especially if it brings you joy.

CHAPTER 21
Voice

What you say is often secondary to how you say it.

There is no getting around the fact that we're judged by our ability to communicate verbally. Many good ideas and thoughts from someone with speech difficulties are not always heard or recognized due to a lack of patience or willingness on the part of the listener to let these ideas and thoughts be expressed fully. In our daily rush of "I want it now" and the fast and furious pace of a quick delivery, someone with a neurological disorder is at a disadvantage.

Numerous intelligent individuals—people with superior minds—have bodies that just don't allow them to communicate aloud clearly. Think of acclaimed physicist Stephen Hawking, who is paralyzed by amyotrophic lateral sclerosis and communicates through a speech-generating device.

He's a brilliant intellect and an inspiration for us all. Whether someone's voice is soft and muted or broken and barely intelligible, if the listener makes a judgment or loses interest in what is being said, then content will be missed due to the poor "delivery." The speaker may have valuable input to offer, but be given little or no credit for content. This creates frustration for both sender and receiver. Such is the case of the Parkinsonian and so many people suffering from other types of neurological disorders.

Both Parkinsonians and their listeners need to recognize the quality of the voice needs to be addressed in hopes of improving communication. The solution may be voice training, special technology, or something as simple as avoiding noisy places. Portable voice enhancers may be of assistance. Treatments like Lee Silverman Voice Training (LSVT) and the Parkinson Voice Project (PVP) can be effective if started at the right time. I completed the training and it has made a difference for me. See the Resources section at the back of the book for more information about technology and training.

Always remember, there is a duty upon listeners, as well as speakers, in any conversation. The listener should try to find patience and understand that the speaker is not being difficult by choice. Like anyone else, people with neurological disorders want to be heard and understood.

CHAPTER 22
Trying to Understand PD

"You can't smooth out the surf, but you can learn to ride the waves."—Author unknown

Parkinson's disease is misunderstood because people routinely categorize it as an ailment of the elderly. On occasion, you hear about a celebrity like Michael J. Fox who has the disease or the media decides to pick out a young person as an anomaly. Mostly we hear about people getting PD after the age of sixty.

There are conferences specifically for those with Young-onset PD. Having attended four of these conferences, I am seeing more people like me, in the prime of their lives, people in their twenties, thirties, and forties, being diagnosed with PD.

PD can rob us of our self-worth, dignity, and independence, if we let it. There is a duty placed on us to educate the public about PD because we are ambassadors. Our bodies are slaves to our medication, and even so, we never can be assured of its efficacy. Being prone to extreme stiffness one moment, we may be writhing and flailing uncontrollably the next. Thus, society's peering eyes makes anonymity difficult for us. I very well could have named this book *Mommy, Why Does that Man Move Like That?* because of the many times I've heard young children innocently, and honestly, ask this question while I twist and turn from dyskinesia in a public place.

Uninvited or unwanted, such attention can pain the psyche. Sometimes the unwanted attention is an opportunity for you to educate the unenlightened. This is your chance to teach and bring awareness. It is not uncommon to see stares, gawks, grins, and laughs from voyeurs who watch me. Other people simply ignore me—on purpose—because they do not know how to respond to me. As uncomfortable as it is, the reaction is an understandable human response.

I remember going through a major airport and having three foreign female Transportation Security Administration agents watch me shuffle through the labyrinth of their security gate. The three were giggling as if I were the entertainment for their coffee break. Had I been in a less dicey place, I'd have been able to educate these ladies on how to be a bit more understanding, compassionate, and humane. To laugh at someone else's inability is the truest sign of ignorance.

Not everyone understands, nor is everyone a compassionate human being. We expect our loved ones, friends, associates, and colleagues to understand our struggle with this difficult ailment. We expect them, sometimes, to care. Those who are healthy and untouched by PD are incapable of understanding what we endure with this mysterious and troubling disease. Some don't care to understand. Caring isn't a part of their emotional matrix. Parkinson's challenges us all in different ways. Rarely, if ever, do two PD patients share the exact same symptoms. As much as we'd like for those who are close to us to understand, it just isn't possible.

Part of having a disease is demystifying it. I think it is important to educate yourself and others. Go to conferences. Start a support group. Write about your illness for a newsletter, blog, or local newspaper. Only through education will we see change and have any hope of those not stricken with disease learning to comprehend what it is we deal with on a daily basis.

CHAPTER 23
Take Me for a Ride

Enlighten the uninitiated.

On December 2, 2007, I took a train from New York City to Washington, D.C. I had an encounter with a ticket collector on that train which disturbed me, even as it taught me so much about interacting with people. It's a lesson I hope no other person afflicted with Parkinson's ever has to go through. This incident was eye opening.

My wife, Angela, and I were returning home from a Michael J. Fox Foundation event. New York was dealing with the first snowfall of the season. The hectic pace of the city's rush hour and the challenge of snagging a cab didn't make the morning easy for us. With only limited time to spare, we made it to the station just as the announcer in Penn Station was calling for passengers to board the train. With all the walking, the stress of rushing, and the fact that it was early morning, it was only a matter of time before my medications would soon lose their effectiveness—and they did. As we walked to give our tickets to the Amtrak rep at the escalator going down to the track, I felt the meds turning off. We approached the gate for the train and my wife handed the rep our boarding passes.

"Why are you holding his boarding pass?" the woman snidely asked.

"His hands are full and he has Parkinson's disease," Angela replied.

"Next time, give him his own pass to hold," was her comeback.

This was going to be a great trip.

The frenzy of New York City and travel ramped up our emotions and the whirlwind of sights and sounds only added to the frenetic energy. Angela and I had begun the morning with a silly argument and the rudeness of this lady pushed my wife beyond her emotional edge. We entered the cabin together, but Angela needed some time alone. She went by herself to the café car. Since I wasn't walking well, I sat down in the handicapped seat nearest the door and waited until my meds kicked back in. The ticket collector, a neatly dressed man in his early thirties, came by and said, "You can sit in that seat until someone needs it."

"I have Parkinson's disease," I explained. He looked long and hard at me for a good ten seconds. His face was full of doubt.

"My mom has Parkinson's disease and she has a card!" he answered. You could hear the doubt in his voice. Was I really going to lie about having PD to keep this seat?

"I'm sorry," I replied.

Then he said it—and I'll never forget this, "Can you prove it?"

Prove it? He wanted me to prove it? Was he serious? How come I had never received my official membership card? I didn't have my medical records with me, and so rarely does someone seriously question the legitimacy of my statements about my health that I was stunned. I felt dizzy. He wanted me to prove that I had PD? No one had ever challenged my authenticity as a sick person. How many people would choose to fake having Parkinson's disease? Would I really choose Parkinson's as the illness of choice just to secure a seat on the train? I don't think so.

"I can walk funny for you," I answered, trying to make light of his request. The ticket collector didn't even smile. He was seriously demanding proof that I had Parkinson's disease. I frantically scoured my wallet to find a tattered card that I picked up once at a Parkinson's conference which declares that I have PD in case I am unable to speak. Luckily, I had signed it back then.

The ticket collector checked my driver's license. That was up to date, though it had been unused for many years. For a good five seconds, he stared at my identification with great scrutiny, as if he'd never seen a Virginia driver's license before. Then he compared my signatures from the two documents and with a snap of his wrist, handed them back to me, grudgingly saying, "Okay!"

I had passed his test—oh happy day!

The ticket collector had no remorse or regret for this confrontation. Although his mother and I share a unique bond, this shortsighted man failed to identify how much we have in common.

Ironically, I almost always travel with a laminated letter from my neurologist that confirms that I have Parkinson's. (See "Ask Your Doctor for a 'Health and Travel Document'" on Chapter 8.) I had it made for me just in case anyone at an airport ever questioned my condition. But of course, the one time that I actually needed the letter, I didn't have it with me. My safety letter surely could have ended the hassling and awkward moments a lot faster.

This was Amtrak and this man's mom had Parkinson's—so where was his compassion and understanding, I wonder? Surely, my telling him that I had PD for over twenty years should have placated his distress over my occupying his sacred seat. He wasn't so much ignorant, as rude. The lesson I learned is that I needed to be prepared in public for all encounters whether with law enforcement and security personnel, transportation workers, or someone else. It is important to carry some proof of condition at all times, because you never know when you'll need it.

CHAPTER 24
Travel Tips

Stay flexible and retain your sanity.

Here are ten tips for travelers.

- Keep your pills with you at all times. Make sure you have enough for your trip and a few days extra in case you are delayed or held over.
- Your pills should be in their proper prescribed bottle in case security or anyone who may tend to you is able to easily identify your drug regimen.
- Ask your doctor for a safety letter printed on your doctor's letterhead, like the one we discussed in Chapter 8. The letter may cost you a little extra but it can serve you well as proof of your condition. Make sure your doctor signs and dates it. To preserve it, have it laminated at a local print shop, FedEx Office,

or UPS Store.

- If you have moments where your speech or fluency is affected by your condition, you might want to print a clean, clear, and simple introductory card to explain your out-of-the-ordinary symptoms or related gestures. Keep several information cards in your wallet, and even laminate some for reuse.

- Before you leave home, study the layout of airports and train stations on the Internet so you can see how much walking is involved. If you have mobility or stamina issues; reserve a wheelchair or a courtesy ride to your gate by calling ahead.

- Pack an extra pillbox in case you lose your current one. Make sure your name and cell phone number are on everything, so you may get your medication back if your bags are lost. Make sure your pills are in the carry-on bag and not in the checked luggage in case that gets lost.

- Keep good records and copies of your medical records. Even better, have your records scanned and put on a computer memory stick to be portable and complete.

- If you have balance issues, avoid escalators and stairs. Plan your trip and map out the location of public elevators beforehand. Wear comfortable shoes that provide support and allow for maximum foot and toe flexibility. The freer your feet can flex, the better your step. You may want to take a folding walking stick with you for added support.

- Stay on schedule with your medication. Even

if time zones change, your body is still on a schedule. Closely monitor your regimen. You may want to use a timer, alarm, or scheduler so as not to miss a dose.

CHAPTER 25
PD Defined

The delicate balance of wellness depends on incalculable factors.

What is Parkinson's? This is a question I get all the time. I thought about it and I have an answer.

Parkinson's, at first, is an itch you just can't scratch. It's an irritable suit that is two sizes too small, and it won't come off.

Parkinson's is expecting reliability from your body and mind, and often getting cooperation from neither.

Parkinson's is about planning ahead and re-scheduling at the last minute because the disease got the last say.

Parkinson's is hoping that the planets are aligned just right and your meds, mood, diet, energy level, sleep, and mobility all let you function as you want to, and not as the disease wants you to be.

Parkinson's is finding your hidden self within this altered being that is the disguise PD creates.

Parkinson's is a python-like lead shell that slowly encases your feet and wraps itself around your legs and the rest of your body, making movement feel difficult and restricted.

Parkinson's is a thief that may slowly steal your independence—though sometimes self-composure and a positive outlook can make the difference in maintaining and even slowing its grip.

It is your choice how you deal with this or any illness!

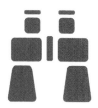

CHAPTER 26
PD Puts Your Life in Focus

Taking the easy way rarely completes the task at hand in a satisfactory manner.

I will not tell you that having Parkinson's disease is a walk in the park. It can dictate your life and clutter your schedule every which way. I have seen it take its toll on many a marriage and family. I have also seen PD bring people together and strengthen family bonds.

How you and your own friends and family deal with your diagnosis will play a large part in how you deal with this illness itself. Some friends are going to be your rocks and will be there when you need them the most. Sadly, some friendships may crumble. Some friends will distance themselves from you. This is the unfortunate reality, but some people can't go beyond a certain limit in their friendships. Some people just cannot accept bad news. Even close friends may decide that in some dark thought that they don't want to watch you go downhill. Your true friends and family will shine, however. Illness, like any big change, can bring out both the best and worst in people.

Generally, you'll have no trouble identifying who is going to stand by you and who will jump ship. You may get a few surprises along the way. It is my belief that my true friends accept me whether I am healthy or ill, and if they don't accept me, then that's just the way it is. There is only so much that we are able to change.

Living ill truly weeds out who in your life are your friends. Disease brings out the personality and authentic character of those around you. For some, there may be an adjustment period, where they, like you, are trying to understand the changes that you're undergoing. Give them time and assistance, if you are ready to do so. Help them to get their arms around what your disease means, as it relates to your friendship. Prepare them for the best and the worst possibilities. Your true friends will accept you in the best light and in your darkest of times. Living ill is not easy. Real friends stick with their friends through the good and the bad. You can only hope that they will be there.

Acceptance is one of the hardest slices of the disease pie to swallow. Accepting that your life is different now, accepting that you are no longer like everyone else, accepting that you're not going to be able to do some of the things that you once loved, accepting that some priorities have changed and others have moved higher up, accepting that every day, hour, moment, and second is precious, and accepting that you are a mortal being. But, you do not have to accept being around people who don't accept you. Let go of unwanted and unnecessary negative energy. Any way you slice it, you certainly don't want to be surrounded by people who cannot accept you and your condition.

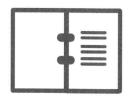

CHAPTER 27
It's Only a Matter of Time

"Time is but the stream I go a-fishing in."
—Henry David Thoreau

W hether you see time as a naturally occur-
ring force, a convention of man, or just
the unforeseeable perpetuator of those
unwanted wrinkles and age-related developments,
there is no denying that time dictates our lives
more than any one influence. Clocks, watches,
calendars, day planners, computers, tablets, and
smart phones all contribute to how well or poorly we navigate our daily lives and human interactions. Tools of organization and predictability add
order and structure to a world that is far beyond
predictable and nowhere near orderly.

Time ultimately robs us of our abilities. As best
as we can understand, the length of our lives is finite. The perpetual cycling of time also takes our

capabilities away from us, as Parkinson's disease can be progressive. But time occasionally gives back to us as well. Sometimes it heals us. So in fact, there is no telling where time will lead us. All we know is that there are 1440 minutes in a day. It is our choice what we do with them.

For someone with PD, there is no knowing when or how long your medicines are going to work or last. Ours is a disease that forces patience and relinquishing of control. Stress, lack of sleep, commotion, being rushed, the daily hustle and bustle, and the presence of a crowd, effect even the healthiest of people. Someone with a neurological disorder like PD is most likely unable to function well when exposed to one or more of these stressors. The harder we push, the harder the stress and negativity that comes with our need for rapid results pushes back on us. Some of us are predisposed to accommodate a frenzied pace, but many of us, if not most, are not. Are you on a collision course for neurological disaster from stress and pressure?

There was a time when society believed that good things come to those who wait and patience is a virtue. Now, fast is considered best. Fast has become the staple of the Western diet, and a desire for speed is quickly invading the rest of the world. Speed is king. In a world of constant flux, on-demand gratification, and throwaway everything, it is only natural to wonder if the affliction of PD is the result of the demands and taxing of a weakened immune system.

It is so easy to miss the little lessons that are thrown our way, every day. Maybe the journey is as important as the destination.

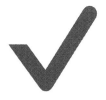

CHAPTER 28
Is Everything All Right?

I can handle the rain; it's the hail that hurts.

Restaurants can be a wonderful place: You tell them what you want and they bring it to you. Restaurants are more spiritual than most of us would think. A sign out front of one of my favorite cafés read, "Today's Special." This led me to think, isn't every day special?

I went into the café to sit down. My waitress, Beth, a bright-eyed and peppy young lady, offered me a beverage and described the bisque of the day. I ordered my drink and entrée.

The food came and Beth delivered my food on the table. Then the usual question came, "Is everything all right?" she asked kindly.

There's an oil crisis, inflation is on the rise, and there is war all over our planet. Oh, and I have Parkinson's disease, I thought, but did not say aloud.

Questions can be insightful tools.

How often do we ask questions that we don't want the answer to? When someone asks how you are doing, do you just say "fine" or should you tell them the truth? Did they really want an honest answer or were they only making idle conversation?

Quantifying how one feels with a progressive and chronic illness is difficult, especially when the other party is unable to understand the various symptoms that accompany the disease. Parkinson's is especially hard to explain to those who don't live with it on a daily basis. Symptoms may come and go, and it can be difficult to determine which symptoms are due to the disease as opposed to being side effects of the medications.

Parkinson's disease and the medicines can play havoc with your emotions, mental clarity, decision making, and cognition. To verbalize any combined physical, mental or cognitive changes is extremely challenging to a stranger. It's tough enough to help a friend or family member to understand, unless they live with you or see you on a daily basis.

KEEPING UP APPEARANCES

For several years of my life, I was embarrassed by who I was and what I was becoming. My dyskinesia was becoming a two-hour workout of uncontrollable shaking and twitching. When I was finished with each episode, I felt as if I'd just run the Boston Marathon. My clothes were soaked in sweat and my hair was mussed from gyration. Dyskinesia came, at times and still may come, at the most inopportune times. This is when Parkinson's draws real unwanted attention. What looks like a dance to some also may resemble a mild type of seizure.

Sure, at first it was embarrassing to be the standout in the crowd. Then I stopped worrying about it so much. After all this time, I am more comfortable than I once was with my dyskinesia. I don't know if I'll ever be totally and completely at ease with the public display of my condition, but I have learned a few tricks that may help you as they have helped me.

- Avoid crowds when possible. Crowds create energy, tension, stress, and noise. People with Parkinson's may be more susceptible to being influenced in a negative way by crowds.
- Learning to time your medications at the right times can make a difference. Talk to your neurologist and pharmacist to see if food sensitivity may influence your medication and if you need to re-schedule your pills.
- Be wary of time-released medicines as they can be hard to time and control for some patients.
- Avoid escalators if you have balance issues.
- I was experiencing a buildup of medication at dinnertime when I was taking time released meds. Dinnertime became unbearable. When I stopped the time released meds, and switched to the regular release pills, cutting these in half and taking a half a pill six times a day instead of three times, the results were impressive! No more dinnertime dyskinesia. I seemed to experience, and still do experience, a more level dose of dopamine in my system with this regimen.
- Closing my eyes and meditating can slow or

stop the uncontrolled movement. Too many thoughts and feelings rushing in can bring on an episode, so remaining calm is imperative.

- If you are on an agonist, such as Mirapex or Requip, and are experiencing dystonia (severe involuntary muscular cramping), it could be a side effect from the drug. Talk to your neurologist.

- If you have access to a neurologist who is a movement disorders specialist, I recommend getting a consultation about any symptoms of dystonia or dyskinesia.

- For PD-related voice symptoms, consult an accredited PD speech pathologist that knows Parkinson's (see Resources).

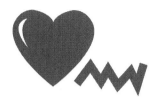

CHAPTER 29
Positive Daily Living

"Finish each day and be done with it. You have done what you could. Some blunders and absurdities no doubt crept in; forget them as soon as you can. Tomorrow is a new day; begin it well and serenely and with too high a spirit to be cumbered with your old nonsense."—Ralph Waldo Emerson

Too often we let others define us, whether for the positive or the negative. Only you as an individual know who you are. You are not defined by what you own, what you buy, or what you say, but by what you think and do, and whom you help, and how. Peace comes in knowing who you are.

Key individuals in our lives have a dramatic influence on how we face adversity. It is therefore vital that you surround yourself with positive people who will support you with an optimistic attitude. In a negative world, it is easy to turn negative. Those with a better attitude will do better in meeting the challenges of living with PD. I firmly believe this to be the case.

POSITIVE AFFIRMATION
Although I am ill, I will focus on the life granted to me. Today is mine to do with as I please. I can make it a day like no other. My perception of the world around me plays an important role in my well-being. Positive attitude starts with a conscious choice to change for the better.

SIMPLE PLEASURES
Illness reminds us that the simple pleasures are the best and should be savored. Whether it's a crisp fall apple, a hot shower, or a breathtaking vista, what most people take for granted is really a precious gift. Disease offers a unique perspective—one that many are not privy to.

Rarely do we live in the moment. Either we reflect on our past or look to the future. We must try as best as we can to savor the present as we better our vision of our condition.

THE POWER OF A POSITIVE ATTITUDE
As callous, awkward, and bizarre as this may sound, illness can often bring out the very best in us. We all digest the reality of living with illness in an unpredictable way. Each of us must be prepared for

the worst, but remain strong and hopeful for the best! Remaining hopeful is key.

In grammar school, I had a teacher who constantly harped on the word "attitude." "It's all about your attitude," he used to say in a strong Southern drawl. I would emulate him behind his back and snicker at his sharp focus on attitude. It took getting sick for me to find the importance of humility, compassion, and acceptance. As my attitude shifted, so did my perspective.

Attitude to me means being realistic, making the best of your situation, and making a positive impact on others. Be it educating, support, inspiration, or comforting, I find it helpful assisting others. I am fortunate, as a person living with a chronic disease. I know this even at forty-five and living with Parkinson's—and having had it now for most of my life, I am grateful and do not take it lightly that I am in good health in spite of PD. I do not have to face a series of painful surgeries, or suffer from chronic pain.

Attitude, attitude, attitude. It sounds funny and cliché, but it is so true. A good attitude will serve you well. Not only will the people with you find you more pleasant to be with, but you also will find you feel better. Positive attitudes promote healing. Having goals is a focus for your survival. Hone in on your purpose and what you need to do to achieve that purpose. As Wayne Dyer says, "Don't die with your music still in you." Do what you can, while you can!

What we say, think, watch or even sing in the shower weighs an impact on us all. If we aren't careful or observant, we can get in the traps of letting people and daily situations zap us of our strength and health. Staying connected to people keeps us healthy. A friend told me how he feared the death of his eighty-seven-year old mother because he knew that his ninety-three-year old father would be sure to follow quickly. Whether or not we like it, we are connected.

I have been ill for so long that I find it difficult to recall the days when I was disease free. Disease becomes part of you. It can alter your personality and worldly perceptions. On occasion, my wife reminds me that she does not know what I was like before Parkinson's. Fragmented pieces of my youth come back sporadically and intermittently, but mainly that part of me is a faint memory. It does me no good to dwell on what is gone or regret on what is lost.

Earle Nightingale used to tell a poignant story about a man searching the world for diamonds. He traveled the world and looked everywhere, or so he thought. Once back home, however, he went out to his backyard only to discover that diamonds had been buried there the entire time. The moral of the story is that we take the good things in our lives for granted and often we have what we need if we just open our eyes.

Diamonds in your life could symbolize the people in your life, the work you do, or the dreams you have. These diamonds are not always obvious at first, but with a hard look we can recognize the positive aspects of our lives.

FORGIVENESS AND OTHER SPIRITUAL PRACTICES
Forgiveness is setting aside our response to past

wrongs that we feel have been inflicted upon us. To notice a real, positive transformation in our attitudes, we must begin to make forgiveness a daily practice. We must also practice kindness. Kind intentions have spiritual value, but kind actions have real meaning. Sometimes, kind acts and forgiveness feel like sacrifices. If so, remember that while sacrifice often seems difficult, it is a sign of faithfulness to principle and our beliefs, nonetheless.

Love is faith, trust, and generosity all in one, without placing conditions on another being. Giving is providing others with aid unconditionally. Trust is giving more than we have and expecting nothing in return. Compassion is putting the needs and feelings of other people and life forms ahead of our own. Patience is respecting the time of others. Real listening is the act of taking meaning and substance from others without premature judgment, criticism, or bias.

REDUCE EXPOSURE TO NEGATIVE INFLUENCES FROM THE CULTURE AT LARGE

You have a choice. From the time when you awaken to the time you lay your head back on the pillow, you can choose to take either a positive or a tainted view on life.

Oil spills, terrorism, earthquakes, tragedy, mudslides, Hollywood, injustice, hate, cruelty, death, crisis, and destruction! This is what makes up the content of our television news programs as well as a large percentage of what we read in the newspaper and what we hear on the radio. Sad and scary news sells well at the box office and in print. In addition to Stephen King, Dean Koontz, and

Wes Craven are just a few of the novelists cashing in on our human attraction to being scared.

If one has Parkinson's disease or any other chronic illness, it is my opinion that one has enough to contend with already and would benefit from eliminating or at least drastically reducing one's exposure to as many negative influences as possible. I, for one, need not invite fear into my life.

Do we really need to add negativity and additional fear to our lives? Our job should be to keep hope alive by seeking and finding the positive in each day, and improving the quality of life of ourselves and fellow humans, as well as the creatures inhabiting this planet. Battling an illness of any kind is a daunting task. For some of us, being ill is a full-time job. Escapism is therefore only natural. Sometimes, when reality isn't what we need, we choose to turn things in our lives off and turn on the entertainment. But, maybe rather than escaping, the answer is to face the issue or problem head-on and create a better reality for ourselves.

Negative outside forces can weaken our immune system. Keeping a positive perspective and fending off energy-draining influences that have nothing to do with you or your condition may be of benefit to you, mentally, physically, and spiritually. Here is a list of things that may help keep you on track in maintaining a positive perspective.

- Take a break from your intake of negative news for a while, and limit your doses of non-essential information from other sources.
- Do something to help someone else.
- Read, write, or listen to something that uplifts you.

- Stay in touch with friends and keep a network of support.
- Join or start a support group.
- Listen to upbeat music.
- Appreciate the love of family, friends, and pets. No pet? Go to an animal shelter and adopt your new best buddy!
- Don't succumb to stress!
- Focus on what you are still capable of doing—and continue employing these capabilities—and do not focus on that which you can't do.
- Seek out a passion or hobby, if you don't already have one. (Be realistic of your limitations, but go outside your current knowledge base.)
- Learn and practice stress-relief techniques and meditation.
- You have a choice how you treat yourself and others. Starting the day with a smile and a positive perspective brightens your day and those you meet.
- Plan as much as you can, but remain flexible and be prepared for changes. Book some events, such as outings, a backyard picnic, a game night, a favorite movie or a favorite meal, so you have something to look forward to, but alter plans as needed.
- Set realistic goals that will give you a sense of accomplishment. Start small and work your way up.
- Don't be too hard on yourself when you falter. Everyone has tough days.
- Keep inspired. Amazing events are happening all around us all the time. See the morning sunrise. Watch the night sky. Observe.

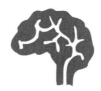

CHAPTER 30
The Mental Side of Parkinson's

An overactive mind can't be calm and peaceful. A slower mind may want exercise. Balance the two extremes.

With any illness, symptoms periodically crop up that may be related to aging, a new unrelated condition, a medicine, or your disease. For some people, Parkinson's disease predominantly manifests as a mental condition while showing few or no other notable symptoms. I have seen Parkinson's that presents itself in this way destroy marriages, cause fights for no reason, incite angry or resentful children, and break up families.

Even as someone with Parkinson's disease, who understands this issue, I came close to losing my temper when a friend with PD offered me a ride to an event and then forgot to pick me up. As he put it, "I'm not firing on all cylinders today." I have heard countless stories of Parkies overcooking and burning foods, placing forbidden objects in the microwave, putting the milk in a cupboard, or demonstrating confusion, as well as causing confusion and frustration for those close to them.

The brain, like any other muscle, functions best when it is exercised and not overtaxed. A person with Parkinson's disease may (but does not always) process thoughts and ideas more slowly than an average person. Some of us are more prone to confusion than others, but all of us could benefit from efforts to maintain and improve our mental acuity as we age.

The following suggestions are designed for PD patients hoping to improve their cognition:

- Establish a daily regimen of mental challenges, activities like doing Sudoku puzzles, matching games, and crossword puzzles, writing, reading, studying vocabulary, taking trivia tests, and playing board games like chess, checkers, or computer games, like Brain Age on the Nintendo handheld and Wii. Some of these games and puzzles are solo exercises; others can be done along with a care partner.
- Watch game shows and play games that make you think and use memory. Jeopardy, for instance, is great for recall.
- Drink coffee or caffeinated teas. I have noticed that caffeine speeds up my absorption when I need to get moving quickly.
- Limiting your protein intake when you're on Sinemet or L-dopa may prolong the effectiveness of the drug. Some days, I find that if

I eat very little, my meds work better.

- Meditate. Meditation is so important for Parkinson's patients. When I meditate (which is not nearly enough), I see a positive change in my thought process and overall well-being. Check out your local yoga studio for classes to teach you how to meditate or look for one of the many audios and videos that are for sale (see the Resources section).
- Staying hydrated and eating a diet rich in healthy fruits and vegetables may help. As I am neither a dietician nor a nutritionist, I strongly suggest that you seek the advice of an expert who understands Parkinson's or consult a book or trustworthy website. (See the Resources section for suggestions.)
- Stress must be contained or reduced to the best of your ability to preserve mental health as well as physical health.
- Get your rest. Sleep is an important component to staying sharp and alert.
- Talking about cognitive issues with other Parkinsonians can be cathartic.
- Seek professional help. You may want to ask your physician or neurologist for the name of a mental health professional who knows about cognitive issues relating to Parkinson's.

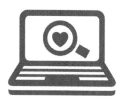

CHAPTER 31
Adapting

"Every exit is an entry somewhere else."—Tom Stoppard

At the time of this writing, I am forty-five years old and have had symptoms of Parkinson's disease since I was seventeen. I've had plenty of time to study this illness and put it in perspective. I would be lying if I were to say, "PD doesn't change your life." Sure, it changes your plans. But I'm not lying when I say it doesn't have to ruin your life.

I meet hundreds of people with PD a year. Most young-onset patients like me accept that their lives must change and that they need to find good medical care. Many older newly diagnosed patients tell me how they had plans and now those plans have changed.

Nothing in our lives is for certain. Whether or not you are healthy, the one certainty is that things change. Plans change. The more flexible we are, the easier it is to adapt to change. As much as we'd like to believe that we're in control of our lives, circumstances outside of our control come about on occasion and when they do we're once again forced to adapt.

Adapting does not mean you stop growing and learning. Transition is a natural process that we need not fight. Taking on this transition with a thirst for knowledge and a desire to improve yourself in mind, body, and spirit, will serve you well.

Try weeding out stressors in your life that deter from your peace of mind. Negative interruptions bombard our minds, from billboards, emails, and talk radio, to television news and other distractions, which upset our calm. Today, try limiting some of these outside influences and see what happens.

CHAPTER 32
It's a Fast-paced World

"There's more to life than increasing its speed"
—Mahatma Gandhi

We live in a world of "faster is better". We demand faster food service, information and news, data/technology, and most everything else. In a society expecting speed and instant gratification, someone with Parkinson's disease or another neurological disorder is at a distinct disadvantage. When time is considered money and faster is better, the individual with PD suffers because he or she may lack the ability to move into fifth gear. In a fast-paced world a person with PD faces the challenge of learning true patience and the ability to learn to live in the moment.

Part of living with PD is practicing acceptance. Acceptance does not mean that you won't continue to seek to better yourself or find better therapies for your condition; it means accepting that you are different and finding comfort in your own skin. Finding the balance in life is a constant challenge. When illness is involved, if it's not put into perspective, it can compound the stress and anxiety of basic daily living with which everyone has to cope.

Coming to grips with your illness may take time and effort. In many cases it may seem impossible, but it isn't. Seek out the part of you that is able to navigate the inner workings of your mind, body, and soul (or spirit) to realize that although this is a challenge, it is one that you can meet. We are stronger and more capable than we know. Adversity can bring out the very best in us and release strengths that we forgot we ever had.

Part of accepting an illness is keeping up the necessary search for relief of symptoms through proper nutrition, exercise, medical care, good drug management, and having a willingness to explore non-invasive complementary therapies that may potentially improve your condition. An open and flexible mind may serve you well in seeking solutions for your condition.

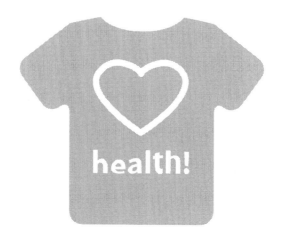

PART THREE

Support Groups and Relationships

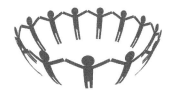

CHAPTER 33
The Joy of
Support Groups

An inspiring word is like a spark,
It gives us strength and lights the dark.
Words offer hope when there is none,
Aiding some to walk and some to run.

For the majority of my years with Parkinson's disease, I was anti-support group. My reasoning (or lack thereof) came from my few sporadic encounters with peer groups in which participants were completely focused on their problems. Many seemed to prefer complaining to helping each other explore solutions. Some patients and care partners in those groups obviously wanted to vent their frustration at being at the mercy of Parkinson's disease, robbed of their freedom of movement and voice. I was looking for camaraderie and proactive solutions.

Rarely, did I get satisfaction of my desires for

support. I don't blame the leaders or the groups I attended. The meetings just weren't run the way I personally hoped they would be and the patients in those groups just weren't looking for my type of meeting.

I had never started a support group. There wasn't a support group in our town and I wanted to connect with peers. With the support of my wife, Angela, we decided to start one. The first meeting of the Fairfax City Parkinson's Disease Support Group began with two guests. It only takes two people to make a support group. You and someone else. Our group meetings can now range from an attendance of twelve to forty members depending on the particular evening, the weather, and the time of year.

Initially, we took the best aspects of the few support group meetings we'd visited over the years and put our own spin on them to develop a format for the support group meetings we facilitated. Since the inception of the group, however, so much time has passed that our core members now know how to keep the conversation and heartbeat of the group pumping, leaving little for us to facilitate anymore. The spirit of the group seems to pass from member to member during our sessions. The group shares knowledge of what is working for them, what isn't working and what to try, and new discoveries that may add to our quality of life. Rarely, if ever, do people talk about feeling sorry for themselves. When they do, our group uplifts them and helps them get back on track by the meeting's end.

My misconception that attending a support

group was a sign of weakness, depressing, a waste of time, and a big pity party was permanently erased from my mind once I discovered that what most people really want from a support group is to:

- Be heard and understood by others like themselves.
- A safe place to be themselves.
- Share their stories in order to teach, help, and inspire others.
- To listen to other people's stories and be inspired by them.
- Cast off the feeling of "being different." For just a few hours, members of the group can be different together!
- Learn about other doctors, referrals, and who is taking certain medications and how they are working.
- A chance to laugh and share your emotions.
- Know that whatever is said is in strict confidence of the group.

Ideally, a PD support group is meant to empower its participants with information, options, and an understanding that the Parkinson's community is just that, a community.

STARTING A SUPPORT GROUP
Support groups can be a place for people to commiserate, but they are also a place to connect and uplift. PD groups give participants an opportunity to learn, to be motivated, and to come away with new strategies for how they might live better with Parkinson's. These meetings are great places

to share resources, such as the names of doctors, services, books and apps. Some support groups are instant successes and others take delicate pruning of the agenda and of the participants to get them running just right. Every support group is an ever-evolving entity, as it rotates in new, as well as longer-standing, members.

I have seen Parkinson's disease support group members range from the ages of twenty-five to seventy-five. A support group binds everyone in that meeting for a unified purpose that transcends all cultural or social labels. Rich or poor, famous or not, each person is there to learn, share, educate, laugh, strategize, congregate, and gain a new perspective.

My vision for a support group came from what I selfishly needed. I wanted to develop a safe and welcoming environment where the group felt comfortable to be at ease enough for two hours to be themselves. I saw this support group as an opportunity to develop an authentic meaningful dialogue between Parkies and their care partners, as well as each other. I take great joy and no credit for the amazing transitions that I continuously see in our group's members. Once quiet members, who formerly kept to themselves or had little or nothing to say, now take the initiative to embrace new members in need and they are always willing to add thoughtful and meaningful commentary. Watching the group grow and take shape has been a labor of love.

On the evening of our inaugural meeting, Angela and I really had no idea how many people to expect. It was a cold, damp March night and

I was skeptical anyone would come. Much to my amazement, one couple actually showed up. I am so proud to say that they are our dearest of friends today and have remained friends, even after all these years.

SUPPORT GROUPS ARE WHAT YOU MAKE THEM

There is no denying that Parkinson's disease is an awful and debilitating illness that makes life much more challenging. Sometimes, therefore, whether or not we like to admit it, we need help. A support group can be an excellent way of receiving the help that you seek.

As someone who used to shun support groups, I decided that I would develop my own style of group. I wanted a group where people could come to feel empowered and educated. A support group shouldn't leave you feeling helpless, alone, or without hope. Our group shares information about new developments in the world of PD, as well as describing what is and isn't working for each of us. Often members suggest something another member could try or suggest ways to "tweak" a symptom that may be the individual hadn't considered. In my mind, this is the model of the kind of support group that can really benefit both a Parkinsonian and his or her care partner.

Here are some ways of running a support group that empowers its participants. Commit to:
- Educating each other and offering possible alternative solutions. This provides an opportunity for everyone involved to change his or her situation for the better.
- Maintaining a positive and hopeful spin on

your comments. This not only keeps the meetings upbeat, it also can make for a more united and cohesive group.

- Sharing doctor information. Other Parkies can be one of the best, most reliable sources of information if you're trying to find the right general practitioner or neurologist.
- Attending. Sometimes just going to a support group meeting reminds you that you have more options in your life than you thought.

Remember, a support group is what the members make it. Like any group, the members keep the group alive. With care and gentle adjustment from leaders to keep the meetings on track, a support group meeting can be a beneficial tool to contribute to personal healing. Illness is a setback, but it is not the end. Although preparing for the unknown can be frightening, knowing you are not alone helps. Confiding in those with similar ailments can be comforting and cathartic. Find or start a support group in your area, and run it the way you feel it should be run.

CHAPTER 34
Relationships Inside and Out

Time may not heal all wounds, for not all wounds are meant to heal.
Scars can be helpful reminders of past experiences.

Build a network of friends and support. Our truest friends and others who care about us will always stand beside us when they're needed most. Keeping social and maintaining your relationships, as best as you can, will help keep your social network active and provide a foundation for this type of support and assistance. Do not forget that there are other reasons for friendships besides support, things such as the pleasure of connection and belonging, sharing interests and hobbies with likeminded people, and the joy of pure fun.

Some people choose to search the depths of

our planet's oceans. Others strive to seek out outer space or the peaks of Everest. It is often said that life is not about the destination as much as the journey. As people with Parkinson's disease and their care partners, we are on a mutual journey of unity, understanding, compassion, and, ultimately, a cure. We are unified by a common cause: Parkinson's disease.

The amazing community of active, vibrant people from across the globe who've been brought together by this common thread is inspiring. Though we're all so different, we are very much alike.

Don't shy away from help if it is available to you. Although you wouldn't want to overuse, or abuse, a friend's good will and resources that are offered to you, if you need assistance in some manner, you should definitely ask for it. By building and maintaining your social network you can drastically increase the number and kind of options available to you.

Some of my relationships have remained solid over the years while I have seen others fade away. I know some friends are unwilling or unable to deal with my changes as my Parkinson's may progress, and I accept that decision. Maybe they are fearful (or defiant) of facing their own vulnerability and mortality. It can be difficult to see people we care about change right before us. For whatever reason, my relationships have changed over time, as has my perspective.

SOLITUDE VS. ALIENATION
Solitude has a place in our lives as much as being social does. Being alone is appropriate when

we find it necessary to discharge emotions or regroup, or to digest thoughts and feelings, but we must beware that we don't remove ourselves completely from the strength of people who can help us if we do retreat. Whether you are a Parkinsonian, a care partner, or a concerned loved one, cutting ties to the outside world can lead to devastating consequences, such as alienation. That isn't it good for anyone involved.

Don't expect everyone to understand Parkinson's. When I was first diagnosed at twenty-three, I admit that the diagnosis came as a relief. What I had convinced myself was a terminally malignant brain tumor turned out to be a chronic deficiency of the neurotransmitter dopamine. That didn't sound so bad. Sure, PD is supposedly degenerative and rarely do PD patients get better over time, but it wasn't a death sentence. I will say I haven't changed my medication for several years. I am lucky and fortunate that my symptoms have shown a slow progression.

We expect our loved ones, friends, associates, and colleagues to understand our struggle with this difficult ailment. Parkinson's challenges us all in different ways. Rarely, if ever, do two PD patients share the exact same symptoms as each other. Those who are healthy and untouched by PD are incapable of understanding what it is that we endure with this mysterious and troubling disease. As much as we would like for those who are close to us to understand what it is that we are going through, it just isn't possible.

Feeling sorry for ourselves is human and only natural upon occasion. When thoughts and/or feelings of sadness arise, remember the moments of your life that genuinely made you happy. Talk to a friend or write about the times of your life and try to remember the joy. Bask in your experiences and accomplishments. Your life is not over, it has simply changed. For now, you must accept your body's changes and stay as strong and as vigilant as you can.

If you think you might be clinically depressed, because your feelings of sadness are deep and have been going on for an extended period of time, or you are feeling hopeless and your sleep, energy, and appetite are being disrupted, you should consult a medical professional.

IT'S THE LITTLE THINGS

One of the loneliest feelings results from experiences with people who are close to us and yet are unable, or unwilling, to accept the nuances of our disease. They either forget the nagging side effects of our meds or misinterpret unrelated physical and mental actions as being drug-related or disease-related even when they are not.

I'd like to think that my identity, albeit altered by illness, isn't dominated by the stranglehold of my PD symptoms, but since PD has played a dominant role in my life for over twenty years, I must expect my behavior and personality to reflect this reality.

Sometimes stress causes my emotions to erupt. *Is it my disease, the meds, or me? I wonder. How can I really know where I end and the disease starts? Are we separate entities or is there an inescapable melding of the body and illness that comes with chronic illness?*

Questions worth considering.

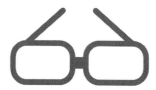

CHAPTER 35
Maintaining
Perspective

Listen. Watch. Be present.

For several months, I counseled a close friend who was going through a messy, vicious divorce. His wife, after ten years, two kids, a mortgage, and large debt, decided she hadn't loved him for over three years. He gradually transitioned from being a heartbroken husband to an angry, vindictive vigilante. Over three months of marathon phone calls, my good friend never asked how my family and I were doing. In his defense, it was a difficult time.

Late one July evening, my friend phoned during a late supper to describe his soon-to-be-ex-wife's obsession with buying a new car that she couldn't afford. "My life is over," I heard him say.

"Stewart," I said, "You'll get back on your feet financially in a year, and in a few months you'll be happy again."

He paused, and then asked, "What? What are you talking about?"

I couldn't pass up the opportunity to share something that was going on in my own life and teach him a lesson. Three weeks earlier, I had returned from Florida. I had been visiting my mother there because she was undergoing treatment for cancer.

While packing the day before my parents were supposed to travel, my mom discovered a lump on her breast. Only one month earlier, her routine annual mammogram had failed to uncover this tumor. Even the sonogram her doctor gave her when he examined the lump barely could locate the invasive intruder. After a lumpectomy, thirty stitches, and severe pain, however, a chest x-ray showed three tumors on Mom's lung and one on an adrenal gland. The adrenal was okay, but the lower third of the lung had to go.

When I left her bedside, she was still facing six and a half weeks of radiation and three months of chemotherapy. In the nearly six previous weeks, Mom had gone under the knife and anesthesia five times. I hurt for her, and while some of my friends tried to console me, many others, like my friend Stewart, were too busy or oblivious to ask how she was or how her condition was impacting my life.

CHAPTER 36
Some Things Don't Change, but People Do

"What I am looking for is not out there: It's in me."—Helen Keller

Often those who have known us longest think they know us best. In actuality, the individual that they once knew and characterized early on may not be the person you are now, or who you have been for years. I, for one, once upon a time was an adamant debater, so I was often labeled as "argumentative." As I have aged, while my brain may still question a comment or fact with which it's presented, I have come to realize that conflict often comes with inquisition, so I don't debate as much. Even though I have come to the crossroads of understanding and knowledge, many who claim to know me seem unable to realize that I made a transition in my life.

Labeling and judging others is too easy and just plain wrong. Be it your neighbor, your best buddy, your spouse, or your co-worker, how many times a day do you label, judge, or criticize someone in your life due to a past action or indiscretion that you've failed to forgive and forget?

Family members that don't see you regularly may fail to recognize changes of progress—in fact, they may see only what they want to see. It is quite possible that those who fail to see you as you truly are, are incapable of identifying the progress because they themselves are not capable of moving forward and they are stuck in past issues with you, not because you're stuck.

We all judge and label. How many times a day do you say, "This is the best" or "This is the worst," or "I hate this" but "I love that"? It is ingrained in us to place labels on people, things, and feelings where they just don't belong. Labeling limits the labeler.

Another set of inappropriate and limiting restraints that we put on ourselves is the restriction of associating every action or reaction in the finite category of "good" or "bad." Not all aspects of our lives can be so easily lumped into one or the other. Good and bad are arbitrary place markers that move around and have fleeting states of reality. There can be no good to compare to without the bad, just as one cannot know pleasure without pain. What we label as "good" one day may appear totally different farther down our path. To label someone or something as being "bad" instead of just accepting that he or she is how they are, constrains you.

It is true growth and a step in the right direction to break this norm of thought about the people in our lives. Thoughts uninhibited by expectations, labels, and judgments can improve our daily lives and our relationships.

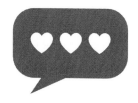

CHAPTER 37
Ten Ways to Improve Your Relationships

"Doing nothing for others is the undoing of ourselves."—Ben Franklin

Here are a few tips for getting along with the people (and creatures) in your life.

- Let go of stupid or insensitive comments, even if someone hurts you. Rise above hurtful talk and poor behavior, and just let it vaporize. Forgive unconditionally.
- Tell the people in your life how much they mean to you. Do something unexpected to demonstrate your love, like come home from work to play with your dog and/or kids, take your spouse out for lunch, or something as simple as a love poem and a hug.

- Call a friend you think of often, but haven't spoken to for awhile. Don't put it off anymore.
- Do at least three kind deeds a day, whether this is complimenting someone, opening a door, or helping a neighbor with his or her computer troubles.
- Share some helpful knowledge with others, either through an email, a post on Facebook or Twitter, a phone call, Skype, or in person.
- Give the animals in your life extra time for affection, play, and grooming. You both will appreciate it.
- Make the first and last thing you say on a voicemail message (and say it slowly and clearly) be your phone number, so that the recipient of the message has easy access to your number.
- The next time you feel angry try replacing that feeling with compassion for someone else.
- A simple smile can brighten your day and another's, too.
- Laugh as much as you can. Make someone else laugh, too.

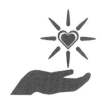

CHAPTER 38
Being Touched
and Intimacy

Everyone can benefit from touch!

To be touched by another human being is a basic necessity. From infancy, we all need love, warmth, and caring. Touch additionally provides people who are ill much-needed attention, a sense of security, and a feeling of acceptance. I have found the sense of touch to be especially therapeutic for me. I have seen it work wonders for many others. Touch can be received through massage, Reiki, or a hug. It doesn't have to be a big thing.

Intimacy is essential. Intimacy can be experienced in a friendship or in a marriage, and it doesn't always have to be sexual. Intimacy is one of the major benefits of a loving relationship.

Touch is healing and intuitive. Just like a mother holds her child to soothe a skinned knee, we all have the ability to reduce pain and ease tension through touch. Whether you get massages, see a chiropractor or osteopath, receive reiki treatments, or engage in other therapies, I encourage the exploration of touch therapies to find out what works best for you.

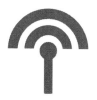

CHAPTER 39
Keeping
Relations Alive

Peace comes in knowing who you are.

Illness shouldn't break up a family. It shouldn't come between spouses. Friendships shouldn't end because a friend is ill. The truth of the matter though is that, sadly, illness tests the family and the spouse, and may put a damper on your interactions with friends. Change of any kind, can be frightening.

Within the dynamics of a marriage or life partnership, this is where communication, understanding, patience, strength, and compassion must be expressed thoroughly. If there was love when you both were healthy, then there ought to be love when either of you is sick. Marriage vows state, "In sickness and in health." Real love means taking care of those that we care about as best and for as long as we can. I will add, as a patient and one who is sensitive to, and aware of caregiver burnout, that caregivers need to be taken care of just as desperately as those of us who are afflicted with PD, in order to assure the health of everyone involved in our households. In many ways, the relationships between friends and family can be similarly strengthened if we treat one another with proper awareness, respect, and appreciation.

Here are some rules of thumb that you and your caregiver may find helpful.

COMMUNICATION

Share your fears with each other and don't hide your feelings. Show your support and love for one another through your personal strength and faith, attending support groups, and getting professional counseling or mentoring. You are stronger than you know. You are not the first people to be tested by what you are going through. This is the time to take stock in your life. Maybe, just maybe, doors close, but when they do, windows open—for a reason.

Stay on top of your situation and seek help as you need it from family, friends, or the local community. Do your research about the services that are available to you locally, statewide, federally, and even internationally. The world is quickly becoming a smaller place thanks to the internet and the sharing of information.

UNDERSTANDING

Common ground isn't always easy to find when one party is in discomfort and the other has a clean bill of health. Just the act of trying to imagine another's challenges can help to put negotiations back on track. Taking the time to listen, observe, and feel another's pain can make tremendous change for bonding and healing.

PATIENCE

Finding that part of you that slows the mind and targets the need on helping one another is essential. Patience is attainable with breath, realization, and commitment.

STRENGTH

I will admit that this may take time, effort, exploration, and even outside assistance. Find what works for you. Maintaining your wits in a crisis is not easy and takes a unique skill set. Dealing with the added stress can take a toll and have impact on those around us. Whether you need a massage, go to the shooting range, break something (a non-dangerous and inexpensive object that provides emotional release), pop bubble wrap (this is reported to be a great stress reliever), work out, sing, or have coffee with a friend, do it. If it helps. Finding what works for you is crucial.

COMPASSION

Loving yourself and someone else is what makes for a complete relationship. It is not egotistical to love oneself. It is necessary, and psychologically healthy. It is of vital importance to maintain your connection with others.

Do your best at doing what you can and surprise yourself. You might just see a change for the better.

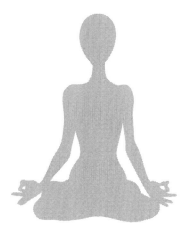

PART FOUR

Reiki, Meditation, and Other Complementary Therapies

CHAPTER 40
Look for
Inspiration
and Answers

"You can't wait for inspiration. You have to go after it with a club."—Jack London

Inspiration may be triggered by almost anyone or anything, at any time. A human interest story may remind you that your life could be worse than it is. An inspiring photo, quote or story can rejuvenate stagnant thought and activate the part of you that says, "If he can do that, then so can I!" Inspiration is all around us. My point here is that you should seek motivation to keep yourself going on the path of building up your health.

NOW IS THE TIME
Good or bad, there will never be a moment exactly like this one. Life's joys sometimes come laced with

devastation, and the unknown can be either energizing or tragic. Perception plays a tremendous role in how each of us chooses to move ahead.

You can choose to make a stand against this disease with grit, gumption, and drive. Maintaining a strong will and determination to heal is a vital step to getting better. Keep your mind open to new possibilities, like complementary and alternative therapies that may become crucial to your mental and physical healing.

Ongoing peace is only attainable for those who seek it. Your willingness to quiet your skeptical mind could be helpful in bringing you peace of mind about your different treatment options. Often listening to your intuition will tell you if a certain modality, such as reiki, qigong, massage, or yoga, may serve you best at a particular time.

Prior to undergoing any irreversible surgery or medical procedure, explore all other opportunities for healing, including alternative therapies and non-invasive treatment modalities that are applicable to your situation. Holistic therapies and energy work such as meditation, juicing, and eliminating or drastically reducing your consumption of meat and processed foods, could make a huge change in how you feel.

Please understand that even if you are sure a therapy is effective and right for you, some practitioners are better than others. Rely on referrals and results from other Parkies. Caution is important when choosing which complementary health care practitioners to select.

STOP AND PAY ATTENTION TO THE SIGNALS

One person's reality is another's paradise or night-mare. The way we perceive our situation sets the rules for our own subjective reality of life. Our emotional wiring, family background, education, life experience, spirituality, and daily insights play a role in how well we process stress and anger. Stress and anger tax brain cells. Taxing our sys-tems to the limits with stress and anger can over-load the body. A large part of living with illness is finding an inner strength and sense of purpose that can propel you forward until you find the an-swers you need. Another substantial component to living successfully, and peacefully, with an ill-ness is accepting yourself. If you refuse to accept what's going on in your mind and body, if you deny that there is something which needs to be taken care of, repercussions such as pain or illness may manifest.

The universe can, will, and does send us a lifeline when we need it, so we must be ready to receive it. If we are unprepared for the lifeline or the message, we may miss a life-changing opportunity.

RESEARCHING YOUR TREATMENT OPTIONS

Your mission with living ill is to thrive and survive. Therefore, take any information you are offered, investigate it thoroughly, dismiss what does not work and keep what does. Your mission is to gath-er together and take advantage of the resources that are available to you to assist you in being as well as you can be. This methodical set of actions could feel slightly overwhelming at first, but you will also ultimately find the management of information to be empowering.

NOW, YOU ARE READY FOR RESEARCH.

You've no doubt searched the Internet using Google, WebMD, the National Institutes of Health website, and probably the websites of several Parkinson's organizations (also see the Resources section at the back of this book). The Internet can be a powerful tool when used wisely or a dangerous weapon when mishandled. Significant errors are often posted online. In this fast-paced information age, we therefore have to be careful to ensure that the data we find on the Web is accurate and has been substantiated. Seek out professional associations, foundations, organizations, support groups, forums, and chat rooms where you can get information about your disease.

Be careful of any complementary therapy you see or hear suggested that has the potential to be harmful in any way or irreversible. That being said, therapies like Reiki, dancing, yoga, boxing, qigong, tai chi, and even interactive video games, are showing great promise for Parkinsonians. These should be considered as long as you don't endanger your health by overdoing it. Obviously boxing is more physically intense than Tai Chi or Reiki. Always consult a medical doctor before making drastic changes in your fitness and health care routine.

WHOSE BODY IS IT?

Over two decades, since my diagnosis with Parkinson's, I do everything more slowly than I once did them. From comprehension to movement, my abilities remain, although they have been altered. Every day is something of a challenge. This isn't a bad thing—it just is. Due to my long experience with PD, I am aware of the importance of keeping both mind and body active. Remaining open to unconventional natural therapies and carefully monitoring my diet has served me well. Although I admit that I could do even better with my fitness and exercise regimen, I do use many of the complementary tools and practices that you'll read about in this part of the book.

Living with Parkinson's disease is like living in a body that doesn't belong to you, as the mind and body develop independent orders of operation. Asked to work in conjunction, the mind often goes in one direction while the body goes in another and does its own thing. When this happens, it can feel challenging. You may even be tempted to give up trying to heal, at times.

What should you do then? Help yourself by remembering to affirm: "I have many purposes. I have a reason to heal for myself and those who care about me. My life has meaning and I will find strength and invigoration in everything I do from now on. Life has new inspiration. This is a challenge and I am willing to accept."

A mantra is a sacred or affirmative statement repeated during a meditation, prayer, or visualization to hold your focus. Use the following mantra to anchor your intention to heal. Many of the chapters in this part of the book will include similar mantras.

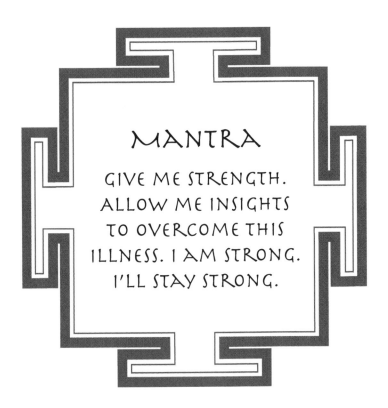

MANTRA

GIVE ME STRENGTH.
ALLOW ME INSIGHTS
TO OVERCOME THIS
ILLNESS. I AM STRONG.
I'LL STAY STRONG.

CHAPTER 41
Finding Reiki

"When you know and respect your own inner nature, you know where you belong."—Benjamin Hoff

I f we are not careful, we allow our healing potential to become restricted by adhering exclusively to conventional Western medicine. I encourage the exploration of alternative solutions as your medicinal needs change over time. Practices such as yoga, reiki, Trager®, massage, essential oils, and a host of other ancient therapies from licensed or certified practitioners (in some cases one or the other, depending on the discipline) and experienced practitioners are options that you might wish to investigate. Those of us living with PD often need help managing side effects of taking conventional medications. Those drugs work better and we can begin, in some cases, to take lower dosages of those drugs, when we are feeling relaxed and fit. With the aid of some Eastern therapies, you may find that you can reduce your meds and side effects. You may see symptoms ease and enjoy the practice.

I can tell you that several of the aforementioned modalities have served me well. I attribute the delay of progression of my PD symptoms to many of these beneficial tools and techniques. The unity of Western medicine with these so-called complementary medicines—which may be defined as therapies that can be used in conjunction with, rather than to replace pharmaceutical drugs and surgery—should be on the frontline of your attack on your disease, along with the options that your healthcare practitioner prescribes. There is a time for new and old styles of medicine to work together, and that time is now: when you need it most!

OPENING MY MIND TO ALTERNATIVES

In 1998, I met a man who became my teacher and a close personal friend. He would teach me the most important tool I have for slowing and possibly reversing the debilitating progression of Parkinson's disease (PD) of which I am familiar.

I had already known the diagnosis of Parkinson's for seven years and had watched how in my late twenties and early thirties this disease took away my abilities and alienated me from friends, and potential friends, who were incapable of looking, or unwilling to look, beyond my illness. There is little understanding as to why some of us get PD at such a young age, or even why any of us get this condition at any stage of life.

By the time I met Gilbert Gallego, M.H.R.D., my life was already becoming limited by PD. I had already chosen, at age thirty, to hang up my car keys and forego driving. While I knew that there were moments when I was able to drive with confidence, I was just as sure that my body was not 100 percent trustworthy. I was not willing to risk my life, or the lives of those I loved, and especially not the lives of the innocent drivers on the road that I could have hurt. I was not going to put others at risk for my own convenience. Besides driving, PD had already forced me to end my love affair with tennis and skiing, two sports that were very dear to me in my early life. As you read on, you will see why I believe that with hope and hard work, maybe, just maybe, I may play tennis, ski, or even drive a car again at some point in the future.

The older I grow, the more I am inclined to believe in destiny. My father had been traveling on business when a minor medical problem flared up. A friend of his suggested a reflexology treatment. The reflexologist he visited also practiced a form of body manipulation called Trager® (also known as psychophysical integration therapy). Finding some relief from the treatment, my father encouraged me to investigate Trager® practitioners in my area. I called the Trager® Society and they referred me to Gilbert. I phoned the number they gave me only to find out that he was moving his current office less than a mile from where I had just moved.

With an open, but cautious mind, I called Gilbert to make an appointment. I had no idea what to expect. For moral support and in the hope that he could help me and somehow help relieve my wife's migraine headaches, I asked Angela to come with me. I had made a 5 p.m. appointment. Angela and I met Gilbert in the lobby of his office. He took us in the treatment room to discuss the rather lengthy set of paperwork that I had completed. He explained his unconventional work as being a "conglomeration" of techniques delivered for what the body requires at the time. Among the techniques he employed, he mentioned Trager®, massage, Reiki, reflexology, and a few other healing modalities. Without too much detail and in hope that he soon writes his own book describing his background, it is safe to say that Reiki gave him his life back.

A retired U.S. Army Colonel, former army ranger, and competitive runner and marathoner for the army, Gilbert collapsed after his last race and lost the use of his legs. No one who examined him at army hospitals or the National Institutes of Health could explain what had happened. What Gilbert now explains as a "mind/body disconnect" had caused his body to shut down. It was Reiki that gave him back his legs and his life.

By now, from listening to him, Angela and I were even more skeptical than before. Hopeful and wanting to believe that this man was the real deal and not a quack would have been difficult for us if he had not seemed so genuine. I asked Angela if she wanted to try Reiki before me, but she told me she had no interest in it. With great anticipation and doubt, I got on the massage table in Gilbert's office for what was my very first Reiki treatment. I was fully clothed, minus only my shoes and belt.

Using only his hands, Gilbert moved around me and shifted my energy. Almost immediately, I relaxed and drifted off to sleep. I had come in walking poorly and was stiff. Ninety minutes later, I came out of the peaceful slumber that I was in to find my limbs more nimble, and my mind and body feeling better than I could remember them being in a very long while.

As I got off the table, I noticed that my whole body felt better. My body was vibrating. I wasn't cured, but I moved more easily. I tried walking and saw noticeable improvement. I felt great and Angela saw a glow in my smile that had been missing. I had gotten something back.

Needless to say, after seeing the positive impact Reiki had on me, Angela was ready to get on the table.

WHAT IS REIKI?

Simply put, Reiki is the transferring of the universal energy that is all around us to renew the depletion of our energy. Reiki helps replenish the body with the life force it is lacking. The person receiving this energy either sits in a chair or lies down on massage table with his or her clothes on. The practitioner giving the treatment lightly touches the receiver.

There is little doubt that human touch is of benefit to our well-being. When I speak of touch here, I mean it in the most caring and compassionate of ways, not just in a sensory or sexual manner. Touch is so therapeutic for pain relief and healing.

If you've never heard of Reiki before, then I

hope that this explanation will intrigue you enough to learn more about what it is and what it does. In the end, I hope I can encourage you to experience the power of Reiki. I think it best to get an understanding of what Reiki is from the words of my dear friend Gilbert, as posted on his website ReikiJinKeiDo.org.

"Reiki is a Japanese word. The Kanji Rei means spirit, and Ki means energy or life force. In essence, Reiki can be interpreted as spiritual or universal life force energy. Reiki is also known as the Usui System of Natural Healing, a very simple technique to aid in the process of healing and many believe that it leads to a path of self-transformation. Reiki was initially brought to the United States by Mrs. Hawayo Takata, a Japanese American, who studied it in Japan in the 1930s.

"Reiki was developed in the early 1900s by a Japanese Shingon Buddhist named Mikao Usui. Master Usui was a well-known scholar and respected healer in Kyoto who undertook an extensive study of healing phenomena as taught through history's greatest spiritual leaders. Through his travels, research, and meditation, he was led to an ancient healing method based on a combination of Buddhist practices performed only by monks and kept as secret knowledge. It is believed that Dr. Usui learned part of this method and received special empowerments and a meditation through which he expanded his understanding of the energy of healing. He spent the rest of his life practicing and teaching this knowledge. One

of his students, a medical practitioner named Dr. Chujiro Hayashi, gave this method a proper structure, which lay people, could practice. Today, this method is now known as 'Reiki.'"

REIKI FOR ME

Sometimes when I work on myself or someone else, my hands get inordinately hot and feel like one magnet pulling toward another magnet. Once in a while, I can actually see the energy move with my eyes. My experience with Reiki has been very positive. Here is what Reiki has done for me and what I have seen it do for others.

- I saw Reiki lower my mother's blood pressure prior to a chemotherapy treatment.
- I have observed tremors and dyskinesia stop.
- I have seen it reduce pain for those experiencing lower back pain and headaches.
- It relaxes those who are experiencing stress and anxiety.

I don't blame you if you are skeptical about any of my observations, but let me ask you this: If Reiki is a non-invasive, non-painful, inexpensive therapy that has the potential to improve your condition, calm your mind, and reduce your stress, then what do you have to lose by trying it a couple of times? I have a strong suspicion that if you seek out a reputable Reiki master (a trained practitioner) and explore what Reiki has to offer, you won't be disappointed.

THE POTENTIAL FOR HEALING IS UNKNOWN

There is a spiritual and a creative side of us that

we set aside in hibernation too often. For no conscious reason, we lose a large part of our identity and our sense of what life is all about. Daily routines, world news, religious cynicism, and the quest for wealth deter us from the true path of healing the planet and ourselves. Each of us knows deep in our minds and souls if our path is the one we are supposed to follow. Life's journey goes far beyond the confines of our mind and body. If logical thinkers accept science, what holds them back from taking the next small step in understanding? Many of life's mysteries are inexplicable. Some may remain so. Others may be revealed in time.

This I do know. Life is about change. It is about personal growth and making transitions within one's life. Kindness, love, and charity are keys to developing true understanding and meaning from life. While our vessel, the human body, holds restrictions on some abilities, there is still far more than we know of what we are capable, including a remarkable capacity to heal.

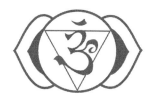

CHAPTER 42
Stress: How
We Can Help
Ourselves

Gilbert A. Gallego, M.H.R.D.

S tress: an all-encompassing word, so common-ly used to depict a variety of modern anxiet-ies and issues. Are the physical, mental, and emotional affects of stress real? Without a doubt, the side effects of modern-day stress are very real to individuals currently living with those stressors.

We all know that stress in itself may be a pos-itive influence, helping to keep us alert and be mentally prepared to live our daily lives whether at home or in the work environment. At the same time, stress can be a negative influence when a person is exposed to continuous challenges with-out some relief, relaxation, or a means of overcoming the stress-induced effects. The medical community believes that stress is linked to six of the leading causes of death in the United States: heart disease, cancer, lung ailments, accidents, cirrhosis of the liver, and suicide.

"Just Do It," the well-known motto of the Nike Corporation, and The Locker Room's slogan, "Think Thin," are conceptually correct. However, the truth is that when a person has the responsibility of taking care of an elderly parent, or is the care partner for someone with cancer or Parkinson's disease and is also working outside the home, the waters muddy very quickly as to how to reduce their own level of stress and still take care of their loved one.

Stressors come in a variety of physical, mental, and emotional issues that can manifest themselves in complex reactions. The complementary or alternative medicine community agrees that the human body is designed to experience stress—if the individual has the means to negate the adverse affects. In my fifteen years of practice as a holistic health practitioner, I rarely find a client that practices well-known methods of stress reduction such as Reiki, yoga, meditation, breathing techniques, qigong, or some type of physical activity with any regularity.

I strongly believe that everyone can benefit from a few minutes of daily, conscious activities that are oriented toward relaxing the body, clearing the mind, and refreshing the spirit. The concepts of Reiki, mindfulness meditation, yoga, or qigong are easy to acquire with minor cost and require small amounts of time—and with great benefits!

> *"I went to the woods because I wished to live deliberately, to front only the essential facts of life and see if I could not learn what it had to teach and not, when I came to die, discover that I had not lived."*
> —Henry David Thoreau, *Walden*

Henry David Thoreau was a proponent for learning to be quiet, for learning to listen to our bodies, to being mindful of the moment, to enjoy each moment as it came to us, of being present and not thinking of yesterday or tomorrow. These concepts of mindfulness meditation can be easily learned from a great meditation teacher, Jon Kabat-Zinn, Ph.D., and his book *Full Catastrophe Living* (Delacorte Press, 1990).

John Kabat-Zinn, in a more recent book, *Coming to Our Senses* (Hyperion, 2006), states: "At the level of the individual person, we know from many studies in the field of mind-body medicine in the past thirty years that it is possible to come to some degree of peace within the body and mind and so find greater health, well-being, happiness, and clarity, even in the midst of great challenges and difficulties."

The second aspect of self-care that I advocate is any style of qigong (pronounced *chi gung*). *Qi* (pronounced *chi*) is the Chinese word for "life energy" and *gong* means "work" or "benefits acquired through personal perseverance and practice." qigong is a very ancient system of gentle, self-healing exercises combined with breathing techniques, which generates a meditative state of mind and is known to enhance and increase one's personal energy field. It is known as a system of slow exercises that involves movements, breathing exercises, various postures, and meditation. These combined aspects of qigong help to increase our natural energy. My personal practice of qigong revolves around those qigong styles as taught by Teacher Li Jun Feng and found in the International Sheng Zhen Society (see Resources section at the back of the book).

The third component is Reiki Jin Kei Do, a therapy that includes concepts from both mindfulness meditation and qigong. Reiki is well known for helping to reduce pain and promote recovery from injuries, illness, disease, and depression. Reiki can also help to maintain a state of inner balance and wellness on all levels of the mind, body, spirit, and emotions. (See the Resources section for additional information regarding Reiki Jin Kei Do.)

Briefly returning to the advice from the Nike

adage, "Just Do It," just do whatever type of Reiki, meditation, qigong, breathing exercises, or yoga you like, remembering it has to be done on a regular basis in order to accumulate any major benefits. We all have an opportunity to enhance our lives by simply acknowledging that we deserve to take a few minutes or a half an hour daily to refresh our mind, body, and spirit by some simple techniques. Good luck!

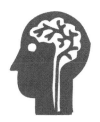

CHAPTER 43
Considering Deep Brain Stimulation (DBS)

Stay informed. Know the risks. Know the benefits.

A dilemma facing many of my friends with Parkinson's disease is the question: When and if I should have deep brain stimulation (DBS) performed?

There is little argument that DBS can make a remarkable and life-altering change in many Parkinsonians' lives. There is also little argument that this invasive surgical treatment is a risky brain surgery that works for reasons that in part still remain a mystery to doctors, their patients, and even the developers of the procedure. Why and how it works is yet to be fully unraveled. The complexities of the human brain hold volumes of unanswered questions and DBS, while it can prove to be of major benefit, it should therefore be carefully appraised by anyone who is considering going forward with this decision.

DBS is portrayed in the media as a panacea. While DBS may make an unquestionable impact on a Parkie's life, it is vitally important to be properly evaluated both physically and psychologically. Before getting it done, be aware of the risks and possibility of infection and lead breaks, and the need for additional minor surgeries every three to five years for battery changes. Also note the fact that even though your dosages of medicine may be reduced after the surgery, you will still need to take medication. I have seen DBS help many people.

Before you elect to undergo what can be a lengthy and invasive procedure, make sure that you haven't overlooked other, non-surgical options that might help delay symptoms: complementary therapies, such as Reiki, yoga, qigong, meditation, and exercise, which can positively impact the body's energy level.

Have you also explored and exhausted the variety of PD medicines?

Talk with numerous people, both locally and around the globe, who have had DBS done to ensure DBS is right for you before you go through with the procedure. Understand the symptoms DBS may help and those functions that it may hinder. Only you know what's best for you.

ALL CHARGED UP
Speaking for myself, I have little doubt that symptoms of neurological disorders like Parkinson's

disease manifest emotionally, possibly being triggered by a physical or chemical jolt to the body. The body's electrical circuitry gets scrambled and disconnects with the circuitry of the mind. If you think of the whole human body as if it were a battery that holds a charge, you will realize that you are dealing with a complex and sometimes fragile network of functions that are all reliant on the body's ability to send out electrical current where it is needed. When the current is weak or broken, problems arise.

"Burn out" is a familiar term that applies to both the body and electrical instruments. When stress, work, lack of sleep, improper diet, depression, and other modern-day lifestyle triggers accumulate, the body, along with the mind, will shut down. It has to, or else it will burn out. Some of us are wired differently (probably through genetics) and are capable of repelling the force of some of these outside triggers, thus evading illness and remaining healthy.

If the body is an energy center in itself and it gets depleted from outside, it only makes sense that the answer to getting the body back in synch is to recharge it from the outside. For thousands of years Eastern medicine has proven that energy work and spiritual practices have real world medical benefits. Slowly, Western medicine is starting to come around and beginning to recognize some of the benefits of Eastern medicine.

As a therapeutic tool, DBS was discovered to be effective by accident. No one knows exactly how it works or why, they only know that electrical signals generated from batteries implanted in the chest cavity, then sent through wires implanted in the brain, can disrupt certain signals going to the brain. This proves to me that we are big power plants that need maintenance.

Energy work is a means of providing maintenance that is mostly free and painless. Time, some dedication and commitment, and some self-exploration may be needed to educate yourself about what works best in addressing your specific symptoms. As unconventional and "new age" as energy work may seem to you, I ask you this: *What do you have to lose in trying one or more of these therapies?*

As overused as the metaphor of the body being compared to an onion is, if you can imagine the moments of our lives, both good and bad, constructing our thoughts, emotions, and overall makeup, then we are what we feel, see, eat, breathe, think, hear, and drink. Delving into the onion and locating the parts that need to be altered may be challenging and may take some time.

There is as much understanding of why energy work makes a difference as why DBS works. The big difference is that energy work has no real risk. It doesn't require drilling in the skull or implanting batteries in the body. DBS is brain surgery and can cost as much as a small house. Luckily, many insurance plans cover the surgery. It would make sense to me that before anyone resorts to the option of implanting hardware in his or her body, the less invasive option is attempted first. If complementary therapies don't work for you and you qualify as a DBS candidate, then you may want to pursue that option, with the agreement of your doctors. Part of getting the most out of your DBS is having the right settings and good programming after your surgery.

CHAPTER 44
The Mind-body Healing Connection

"Happiness is not best achieved by those who seek it directly."—Bertrand Russell

I have a strong hunch that many diseases exist as much in the mind as they do in the body. I have seen people with Parkinson's disease lower their medications and reduce symptoms when they made changes to their lifestyle and living conditions. By eliminating the physical, mental, and emotional triggers that add to stress, the more efficacious their medications become.

HEALING TO A CURE

I have had Parkinson's disease for over two decades. Today I consider myself healed, even if I'm not yet "cured" physically, because of the way I define my "healing," Most of my life has involved coming to the understanding that the mind and body are connected. Words, thoughts, and feelings, which originate in the mind and heart, are the building blocks of our core makeup. Internally, these blocks guide our choices, and externally, they manifest our perception. If you are experiencing a mind-body disconnect, it just means your head and body are not working together.

Illness manifests for a variety of reasons, which may be chemical, genetic, environmental, or other in origin. Sometimes an eruption in emotions can trigger physical disruptions in the body, indicating the mind and body have failed to work in harmony. When the mind and body fail to coordinate, nothing is properly regulated and the body weakens, making it ripe for imbalance.

If we fill our minds with powerful healing beliefs about living in balance with Nature, we can harmonize our heads and hearts. This works, because this world, as we know it, goes far beyond and deeper than the five physical senses of humankind allow us to perceive. Our understanding of the human body, the brain, and much of our planet are yet to be fully explained or understood. There is so much that remains a mystery to science and medicine.

Repeat the following mantra to promote universal healing in your body and mind.

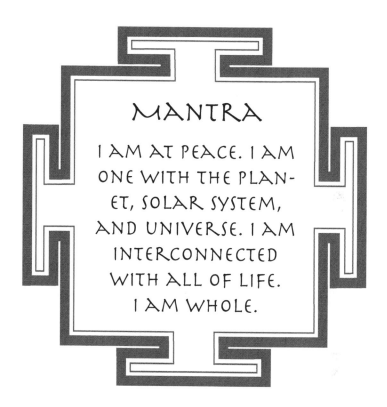

MANTRA

I AM AT PEACE. I AM
ONE WITH THE PLAN-
ET, SOLAR SYSTEM,
AND UNIVERSE. I AM
INTERCONNECTED
WITH ALL OF LIFE.
I AM WHOLE.

THE POWER OF VISUALIZATION AND MEDITATION

Hope is a vital element in preparing your body for its battle with illness. You can develop hope by focusing your mind on getting well and taking charge of your healing process. If you can keep a positive outlook and see yourself improving in your mind, your body may follow.

Visualization and meditation are two powerful tools of focus that you may want to explore to overcome anything that is preventing you from experiencing healing and wellness. Limitations of belief are finite boundaries that we use to restrict our full potential. Opening your mind to new ways of healing can make a tremendous difference in the efficacy of your treatments. The more receptive you are to the energy all around us, the more productive the healing.

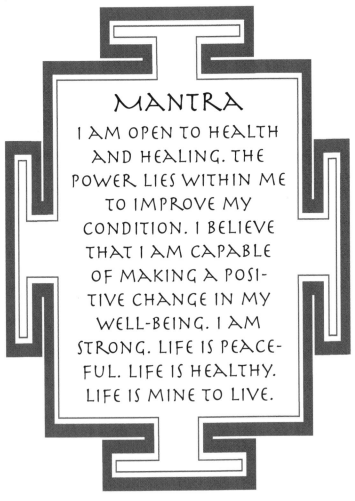

MANTRA

I AM OPEN TO HEALTH AND HEALING. THE POWER LIES WITHIN ME TO IMPROVE MY CONDITION. I BELIEVE THAT I AM CAPABLE OF MAKING A POSITIVE CHANGE IN MY WELL-BEING. I AM STRONG. LIFE IS PEACEFUL. LIFE IS HEALTHY. LIFE IS MINE TO LIVE.

USING MEDITATION AND VISUALIZATION FOR STRESS REDUCTION

Living well with Parkinson's involves learning to deal with stress in our lives. Stress management is essential to preserving your health, so identify and limit or eliminate your exposure to the known triggers in your environment.

Meditation has powerful calming benefits for both mind and body. Take the time to educate yourself at a local yoga studio or Buddhist center about how to do it.

Meditation can be as simple as watching your breath move in and out of your body with gentle awareness. Sit quietly and track the sensations as the air you inhale travels in your nose, down to your lungs, and back out again. Do this for five or ten minutes at a time—or even for a few breaths—and you will be amazed at how deeply restored your body can feel.

JUST LET IT GO!

When a thought or emotion comes up during a meditation and intrudes on your attention, tell yourself: "Just let it go!"

Sure, saying it and the actuality of doing it are different, but it becomes reality the more you do it. Meditation and the acknowledgement of letting go is a practice, and this is the benefit of the practice that comes with continuous use.

So often in our lives we are asked to let go, be it through the loss of a loved one, the breaking of a promise, feeling the impact of an unkind act, the need to release a dream, resentment, guilt, or a deep-seated emotion. Letting go is an ability that takes practice, discipline, and intuition. It also takes timing. Knowing what to keep and what to release sometimes requires us to take a leap of faith into the unknown. It requires bravery.

Whether you hope to shed pounds, bad habits, clutter in your life, resentment, or the past, it is a good practice to remember to let go of what you don't need or doesn't benefit you.

CHAPTER 45
A Simple Healing Visualization

"You have everything you need for complete peace and total happiness right now."—Wayne W. Dyer, Ph.D.

Sit in a comfortable spot where you are able to be quiet and calm, such as a comfortable chair or a pillow on the floor. Once you are settled, close your eyes and take a few deep cleansing breaths, and then begin.

At your own pace, calmly take six to twelve calming breaths. On each full breath, slowly inhale through your nose and then exhale through your mouth. Pull air deep into your lungs before you release it. As you expel the air, feel the stress and tension release from any part of your body that carries pain or stiffness. Put any stresses of the day behind you as best you can during these first six to twelve breaths.

With your eyes still closed, envision a small round golden bead. Pure and golden, the bead shines a healing golden light. The bead reminds you of a shiny pearl, but its amber brilliance radiates from the core rather than from an external light source. Energy pulsates from within the tiny orb. Watch as the bead goes into your third eye, right between your eyebrows. Watch as the bead radiates a warm glow that permeates your entire body. The bead has healing powers, and it has come to energize you and return you to a state of health and well-being.

As the bead emanates energy through your third eye it is seeking out any imbalances that exist in your body. Envision the bead scanning your system for toxins and invasive material. As the bead identifies any unwanted structures, it eliminates them. The healing glow of the bead replenishes the depleted cells and snaps them back to their complete potency.

Once the bead has replenished your body, it begins to fade. After the body has been scanned entirely, the bead will slowly dissolve. To conclude the visualization, take three more deep cleansing breaths, and then open your eyes, feeling cleansed and refreshed.

CHAPTER 46
A Releasing Mantra and Affirmation

"You can clutch the past so tightly to your chest that it leaves your arms too full to embrace the present."—Jan Glidewell

Sit in a comfortable position and close your eyes. Breathe normally. Then begin. The following mantra is appropriate for occasions when negativity is dominating your mental activity.

As you breathe in your next breath, silently affirm: "I am open to healing and making life better with every inhalation."

As you breathe out, silently affirm: "With every exhalation, I release the toxins, anger, hurt, and fear that hold me in this prison of negativity."

Pause for a moment between breaths. As you do, silently affirm: "My mind is a powerful tool that must influence my body to initiate change."

Repeat the mantra for the next several rounds of breathing. Then breathe normally and rest.

This mantra can also be used as an affirmation. Write it on a piece of paper and hang it where you can catch sight of it easily, such as on the wall near your desk or by your bed. Post it by your mirror.

Three times in the morning and three times at night, look into the eyes of your reflection in the mirror and repeat the affirmation out loud. Say it to yourself and also see yourself saying it. This is a powerful way of communicating with your subconscious mind and enrolling it in your mind and body healing.

Make this mantra yours. Change the phrases for your specific situation. This mantra is flexible enough to be molded to what you need, at any particular moment.

CHAPTER 47
A Visualization for Letting Go of the Past

Hope beats uncertainty.

Find a quiet, comfortable place to sit where you won't be disturbed. Close your eyes and breathe. When you feel relaxed, begin your visualization. Imagine you are standing in the middle of a beautiful library. The walls are lined with racks and shelves of books, videos, and journals.

These are the moments and events of your life. Walk to the left and go to a far shelf that has a label on it that reads: "Memories to Keep." Take one of the books off of this shelf and open it to a random page. This is a memory that brings back a pleasant time or event in your life. Allow this memory to replay itself. When you're done, place this book back on the shelf.

Walk to the right and go to a far shelf that reads: "Memories to Discard." The books on this shelf are filled with thoughts and feelings that don't serve you. Each title on this shelf makes up your concerns, fears, anger, or distress. Your energy is robbed by these negative thoughts and feelings, so it is time to get rid of them.

Pick up a book from this shelf of negativity. Rather than opening the book, take it to the corner of the room, where you now notice a vent that reads: "Disposal." Toss the book into the slot and allow yourself to appreciate the feeling as you let go of the thoughts and feelings associated with the memory. Systematically, take each individual book off the shelf in this section of the library and toss it into the disposal slot in the wall. Savor the release that you feel as each book or disturbing memory is destroyed and released from you.

Remember that you can stop whenever you want and take a break. You can come back and dispose of more negative memories, thoughts, and feelings any time it seems like it would be useful.

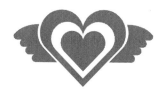

CHAPTER 48
There Are Such Things as Miracles

"Magic is just science that we don't understand yet."—Arthur C. Clarke

L ife on many levels can be difficult and challenging, whether or not we have illness. The added challenge of PD only accentuates the necessity of taking better care of ourselves. It is when we neglect ourselves, or we fail to listen to the cues being presented to us by those around us that something needs our attention, that we miss important and even life-changing messages.

The older I get, the more I am beginning to believe that things happen in life for a reason. My belief is that somewhere in any happening there is a nugget of wisdom to be mined. There may be an appearance of randomness to our lives, while in reality there is an underlying order. Coincidences are often messages of unfinished business that needs to be addressed.

Several years ago, a friend put me in touch with speech-language pathologist, Samantha Elandary. Samantha founded the Parkinson Voice Project, in Dallas, Texas. After I returned from Dallas over seven years ago, I found my voice had improved from just a few days of therapy with Samantha. Time passed and then I ran into her at two different Parkinson's events. At the second event, she told me how her voice program had evolved and invited me to Dallas to see and experience the power of the program. As someone who is fluently challenged at times and speaks publicly, I accepted her offer to improve my speech, fluency, and loudness.

I have been accused of being hyperbolic with my words on several occasions, but what I saw for others as well as me is nothing short of miraculous. People with PD and soft or weak voices were regaining their lost voices. How easily we discount the importance of voice and fail to recognize the self-esteem attached to being heard and understood. The Parkinson Voice Project is fighting to help people with PD regain and maintain their identities and their voices.

What I saw for myself was an increase in volume, improved clarity, and a fluency that I had not seen for years. I saw people at Samantha's center smile with pride as their voices came back and I saw care partners shed tears of joy as their spouses and partners could now be heard.

The old saying that you don't know what you've got until it's gone is true, especially in this case, and for the many of us who won't realize that something needs fixing if we don't pay close attention. For me, I am so grateful to hear such a dramatic change in my speech. Also speaking on behalf of my wife, she is very happy not to need to ask me to repeat myself.

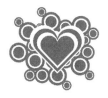

CHAPTER 49
Celebrate Your Life, Not the Parkinson's

"Life itself is your teacher, and you are in a state of constant learning."—Bruce Lee

Someone I respect recently wrote an Op/Ed piece that I felt shone a negative light on people who maintain a positive outlook when dealing with Parkinson's disease. My interpretation of the piece was that it inferred Michael J. Fox was calling himself "lucky," and that anyone who considers himself or herself lucky to have Parkinson's is a "Pollyanna." As I understand the character Pollyanna (in full disclosure, I have not read the book), she went through extreme suffering, but was grateful for what she did have. I see the trait of positivity and optimism as nothing less than admirable. If seeing the glass half full as opposed to half empty, or empty, or even dirty and cracked, is Pollyannaish then please paint me as a Pollyanna, too.

Having lived over twenty years of my life with this challenging illness, I am neither naive nor am I uneducated. I am well aware that this illness robs millions of people around the world of their ability to move, to work, and to function as they choose. The mind seems to get a mind all of its own and neither the mind, nor the body, wants to respond to the other. It was not something I chose to experience. As you know, Parkinson's symptoms of tremor and rigidity appeared in my life at the early age of seventeen and then I spent over six years living without a diagnosis, never knowing what I was dealing with or how fast it might progress.

Was I scared? Sure. Did I feel sorry for myself? Only, after I got booted out of Outward Bound for being considered a health risk to the rest of the hiking party did I feel a real loss. Thankfully though, my dismissal from hiking the rugged mountains of North Carolina, led me to the doctors who finally diagnosed me with Parkinson's disease. Not until years later, did I realize that it took my leaving the group to get diagnosed and move on with my life.

The diagnosis of Parkinson's disease, for most people, can be sheer shock and devastation. For others it can provide a sense of relief.

As a support group leader, a frequent speaker, an advocate for people with Parkinson's, and an attendee of several conferences a year on issues related to Parkinson's disease, I can honestly say that people who keep a positive outlook about dealing with Parkinson's disease, appear to be doing far better with it than those who are less positive.

STAYING POSITIVE IS A CHOICE.
Once I received a diagnosis, I had an idea of what I was up against. The really good news was that as bad as this illness was or seemed to be, there were numerous therapies, medications, exercises, doctors, classes, and support groups out there that could make a difference in my life and help me change my life. Any illness can change how we see ourselves and may get in the way of our perception of who we really are. PD is an opportunity to take a hard look at our lives and observe that maybe a change in lifestyle is in order.

Parkinson's has taught me to appreciate every day, to appreciate and truly be grateful for the good things and the simple pleasures in my life. I didn't choose to spend the majority of my life with Parkinson's disease, but I can choose how I respond to it.

Whether you have Parkinson's disease or you are in perfect health, the realization that a positive outlook not only makes you feel better, but also makes those around you feel better is a powerful realization. Sure, illness throws roadblocks and detours in your path, but that's where your ability to adapt and be creative will come into play. Reducing stress and altering your lifestyle for the better in the areas of diet, exercise, and complementary therapies on top of neurological care can have a tremendous impact on your mood and well-being.

I hope and wish for a cure for all of us. Until the puzzle of Parkinson's disease is solved, I believe the best course of action is to stay informed, take the best care of our bodies and minds as we can, take our meds on time, eat low on the food chain (meaning, eat plants), eat organic, and get our rest. If every day were sunny and warm, could we truly appreciate its loveliness? The balance of life exposes us to pain because without it, there is no knowing pleasure.

Take stock in the fact that people care about you. Focus on the simple things in your life that you can appreciate, like having a comfortable place to sleep, clean air and water, the beauty of nature, and so many gifts of life.

CHAPTER 50
Who Says Parkinsonians Can Only Get Worse?

"If you think a thing is impossible, you'll make it impossible."—Bruce Lee

There is so much gloom and doom on our cable, Internet, wireless, and any other media that I can think of, that it makes me cringe. The bombardment of fearmongers, doomsayers, television news pundits, and Hollywood celebs, may be entertaining but it could be bad for you! Negative energy is simply corrosive and corruptive to the planet and distractive to our healing process.

What you expose your body to (be it water, food, air, sunlight and radiation, stress, chemicals, and unseen forces like negativity, electromagnetic fields, and emotional buildup) will play a vital role in how you cope with and fight off illness. For me, stumbling on Reiki was the key that opened the lock to begin my path to real healing.

I have heard people that know absolutely nothing about Reiki and have no comprehension of "energy work" discount it and call it a "voodoo" therapy. These people really have no idea what they are saying, and it is to these negative ninnies that I say, "Do the research and try it out before you badmouth something that you don't understand." When I was first exposed to Reiki, I discounted it, too, because the thought that using our hands to transfer life force energy for relaxation, stress relief, and potential healing sounded outlandish to me. But when you are ill, taking measures outside the norm are sometimes necessary and justified. Parkinson's disease motivated me to go outside my comfort zone. I'm glad I did.

Anecdotally, I am pleased to report that through Reiki, along with massage, yoga, mild exercise, a hopeful attitude, and a vegetarian diet, I have held steady and reduced my dosage of medication, rather than needing to ramp it up as is expected in Parkinson's disease. The proof is in the results! This has inspired me to give Reiki to other Parkinsonians.

After over a dozen years of practicing Reiki on friends, family, and each other, Angela (who also is a Reiki Master) and I decided to introduce Reiki to the Parkinson's community. With the assistance of eight other Reiki practitioners, we gave a Saturday workshop for twenty-one students that reminded me just what Reiki has done for me. I watched as instant relaxation set in, tremors subsided, muscles released, facial masks washed away, eyes brightened, and lethargy was replaced with energetic zest! If it sounds incredible, well, that's because it was! The feedback from the participants was universally positive.

This was not a clinical research trial, but a shared human experience.

BE SKEPTICAL, BUT STAY OPEN-MINDED

Neurologists and researchers need to step back and look at Parkinson's disease from another perspective. I believe that even though there may be a genetic component, as well as an environmental trigger for PD, there are also emotional, energetic, and psychological components to it that disrupt the unity of the mind and the body. Denial, for instance, is one.

When we refuse to face the obvious or place blame where it is unfounded, problems germinate. Our minds and bodies are sponges that soak up thoughts, feelings, experiences, visions, and impacts. Both the mind and body retain memories. When we fail to acknowledge or accept that we are holding on to unnecessary mental and emotional "baggage," garbage that may be contaminating our energetic systems, problems begin to arise.

For those of us who deny our symptoms, illnesses, or our perspective on own personal health, we fail to realize that there are warning signs being presented. Avoiding a warning sign, be it a tremor, a balance issue, weakness, or any noticeable change in our medical condition should be a wakeup call that there is work to be done. These signs must not be dismissed.

Don't deny denial. Once you overcome denial you can address the issue at hand and begin healing. No doubt, it takes courage, awareness, and trust to admit that you may have an unaddressed physical, mental, or emotional issue. Much of improving our lives is discovering those issues and buffing them out rather than suppressing or storing them. It's called personal growth when we do the work of addressing that which needs addressing.

The first step in breaking denial's hold is taking a hard look at yourself. Don't like what you see? Guess what: You can change it! Accepting that you see something you want to change is a good place to begin. Realizing that there may be work needed (be it physical, psychological, spiritual, or a combination) may be the answer to get you back on the path to optimal health. The sooner that you can make sense of the signals that your body is sending you, and stop ignoring them, the sooner you can help yourself and get better.

For myself, after altering my thought processes, learning Reiki, reducing stress, and realizing certain behaviors that needed tweaking, I have found myself improving over the past several years. My medication has not changed in many years and I continue to get better!

Skeptical? So are some of the Parkinsonians to whom I give Reiki at the PD conferences I attend, but when we're finished, they admit that they feel better than before their Reiki sessions. A simple act of gentle touch makes a world of difference. No pills. No surgery.

AN OPEN MIND MAY LEAD TO HEALING

Parkinson's disease is a disease without any glamour or style. Put a room full of people with PD together and you'll see an array of the same symptoms in a variety of combinations, and you probably won't encounter any two Parkinsonians whose PD is expressed exactly alike.

Parkinson's treatment, for all the research, press, and money that has gone into it, frankly, has not come that far. There are medicines and surgeries to stabilize patients for only so long. These tools may temporarily delay or reduce some symptoms, and help with their voice and mobility. The breakthrough that was being promised twenty-plus years ago, around when I was diagnosed, has yet to come.

If each one of has such a unique case, maybe that means each of us has a unique combination of triggers that set the course for the development of our PD. If that is the case, it just may be within our reach for each of us to find our own cure. As radical as this may sound, I wholeheartedly believe that our bodies, given the right information and regimens, openness to self-discovery, and willingness to change, begin healing themselves. Combined with Western medicine and Eastern therapies, a proper balance of physical and mental conditioning may reverse, or at the very least, improve Parkinson's.

My long journey with Parkinson's has led me down some dead ends but I have also seen successes. In my hunt for healing and therapeutic answers to my condition, I have seen Reiki make the largest impact of any therapy on this disease.

Amazingly, the scientific community shies away from testing this therapy so it is conveniently discounted and dismissed.

GETTING BETTER

After my long history with Parkinson's disease, I am amazed and overjoyed that I have had the ability to consistently improve and show real signs of getting better. I won't tell you that there weren't dips in the road as some of life's roadblocks hit me and my progress deviated. But part of staying focused on my healing is to stay open and flexible in my mind and body.

I've had this illness for most of my life, so I don't expect to get well overnight. My expectations are realistic. My body can only heal so fast. It took me a while to get sick and it'll take some time to get well.

Recently, a major network, I won't say which, other than to say it begins with a "C" and ends in an "S," did a story that I found incomplete, poorly researched, and all-in-all just plain wrong. The story was that a positive attitude does not make a difference when dealing with major illness. Their argument was that modern science has proven that there is no basis for positive thinking to be either a deterrent or a cure for sickness.

I say this report is rubbish. I know people who are better off and showing improvement because they maintain a positive attitude. I am living proof. I think the writer failed to thoroughly research this issue as fully as he or she should have. Even if science has shown that a positive attitude isn't beneficial in fighting illness (which I know is false), who are they to try and dash the hopes of millions of people clinging to the hope of improving their condition? Maybe, just maybe, some reports and supposed "news" should be kept quiet.

I, for one, am staying positive, because it works for me.

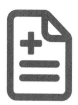

CHAPTER 51
Getting Better

"If anything is sacred, the human body is sacred."
—Walt Whitman

I t is ingrained in most of us not to question the authority of the doctor.

There is no doubt that doctors provide vital and life-saving services, but there are times, especially if you are dealing with life and death situations, that you have the right to question your doctor. If you rely solely on your doctor's advice and treatment you may well be cheating yourself out of ways of improving your condition. You need to be okay in your own skin.

Although they don't announce it, scientists and doctors don't fully understand the total complexity of the human body and brain. It is a lack of understanding that I believe repeals the doctor's presumed right to project into the crystal ball and predict a patient's future outcome.

You must do your part in getting better. Feeling better and getting better begins with a mind shift to knowing that you can get better. The medical community in general seems to think that people with Parkinson's will only get worse, period. They provide little hope for improving our condition and typically add to their prognostications that this illness is both chronic and degenerative. I have yet to hear of a doctor who prescribes hope and positive thinking to his patients.

Positive thinking and hope get people through amazing traumatic events every day. Feats of super-human strength in times of crisis, heroism under severe pressure, survival under extreme conditions, and the ability to push the body even beyond the breaking point are just some of the unexplained medical phenomenon that science can't fully dissect.

Programming can be as dangerous as it is powerful. When a patient is diagnosed with any illness and the doctor tells a patient that there is "no hope," the negative reinforcement that this produces can have devastating consequences on the patient's whole being. Had the doctor said, "We have no medical answer for your illness at this time, I suggest you investigate other potential therapies that may benefit you that Western culture has yet to embrace," it would be different. Of course, you probably won't hear this from most doctors. Shifting the standard outlook from grim to hopeful could revolutionize medicine and improve the lives of the ill seeking a cure or just a better life. There is power in keeping positive.

HARMONY

The energy that you bring into your home and the character of the people who you surround yourself with play huge roles in your mental and emotional well-being. The food you eat to the location of your home may have an effect on how well you function. What you watch on television or the music you listen to can have a toll on your energy and your household. Almost everything you do can affect you, especially if your system has been compromised.

To change our internal programming can take a lifetime, if we ever succeed. Perfection is the most noble of goals, but it is elusive. There comes a time when we must make peace with our worries and lighten the baggage of youth. Life without harmony adds to stress and can be destructive to our well-being.

TAKE BACK YOUR LIFE

As an advocate for Parkinson's disease (PD) awareness and issues related to this illness for so long, it can, at times, be easy to blur the lines of my identity and the disease itself. Losing one's identity in the haze of illness may be comforting or even natural, but I am not my illness.

Healing begins once you take back those thoughts and feelings that you have relinquished to the disease. It's about not giving in and about making the necessary changes in your life. Somewhere along the way, your mind and body may have not gotten what they needed spiritually or chemically. Now, your body is crying for change and the time has come to listen.

Listening to the mind can come in many forms, including intuition, meditation, or self-discovery. Calming the mind will serve you well on many levels on your road to health and healing. Self-awareness comes through self-care. Once the mind is under control and your focus is clear, pay attention to the body and address issues of concern.

Healing may require discipline and dedication. Devotion to improving your condition is the jumpstart needed for taking back control of your life. If you are truly committed to getting better, you must take time for yourself to focus on improving your condition.

CHAPTER 52
What Are You Willing to Do to Help Yourself?

"Few people are willing to admit that their mind could be responsible for physical problems when it's much easier to place the blame on someone or something else."—Robert C. Fulford, D.O.

How far are you willing to go to help yourself? Would you try a complementary therapy that made little sense to you but may have real benefit? Would you sell your favorite objects to gain back your health? Would you change your diet, your job, and/or your residence to get better? How open is your mind to the investigation of learning to find the answers of your illness and healing yourself?

Whether you have Parkinson's disease, some other ailment, or an issue in your life, there is probably an element in your life that could use improving. I have yet to meet the individual who has been able to manage their daily stress, issues from their past, or their fears without being in need of at least a little assistance.

Today, I can say that I am better now than I was ten years ago. Having had Parkinson's for over twenty years, I see this as remarkable and nearly miraculous. My medications haven't changed for many years and, if they have changed at all, it was a slight reduction in pills rather than an increase. It turns out that I can control almost all of my symptoms thanks to Reiki. I am not at 100 percent but I think I am on a good path.

I don't like the words "chronic," "degenerative," and "incurable," and yet these are the words that label Parkinson's and so many other illnesses. These words offer me nothing but doom and gloom, when what is needed is encouragement for motivation and life change. Hope and direction is often what Parkinsonians need. Sometimes a shift in thinking, perception, outlook, emotions, diet, lifestyle, and openness to healing is enough to make the transition of improving our condition. For myself, gradual improvements took time, energy, dedication, and sacrifice.

Getting better for most people is not going to be a quick and easy fix. However, if you open your mind to explore the possibilities outside of your comfort zone, you may very well find yourself seeing improvements in your overall health sooner than you think.

CHAPTER 53
The Power
of Touch

*Touch is unspoken communication and sharing
energetic compassion.*

Over several decades, whether you know
it or not, Hollywood has subtly exposed
the world to Reiki. Whether it was the film
Starman with Jeff Bridges and Karen Allen, *The
Karate Kid*, The *Matrix*, *Elektra*, *Hellboy*, or any of
the numerous other blockbuster films depicting
the power of human contact, Reiki has been a Hollywood co-star. What appears miraculous on the
big screen is a reality within the grasp of anyone
willing to devote time and energy to his or her
own self growth and awareness.

Reiki is a complementary therapy that incor-
porates the use of universal energy. A trained Reiki practitioner is able to transfer universal energy
through his or her hands and allow that energy to

help assist the recipient. I have personally seen Reiki alleviate pain, lower blood pressure, stop or reduce tremors, calm a person down, and rejuvenate someone who is feeling fatigued.

Explaining Reiki is very much like explaining an emotionally moving photograph, a sunset, a song, or a work of art: You can talk about it all you want, but until you experience it for yourself you cannot truly fathom the raw power that it has to offer.

A standard Reiki session can last anywhere from fifteen minutes to an hour and a half. The recipient either sits in a chair or lies on a massage table, fully clothed, as the practitioner lightly touches the energetic centers of the body. People will usually fall into a deep, refreshing sleep when they are being given Reiki and wake feeling better than when they arrived.

I was a skeptic thirteen years ago, but then I tried it. Since then, I have taken classes and worked on hundreds of clients and seen astounding results. I am now a Reiki Master and I continue to learn. For me, Reiki has given me back parts of my life. According to the conventional medical community, Parkinson's patients, especially someone like me who has had PD for over twenty years, aren't supposed to get better. Reiki is the only explanation for why I'm seeing my condition reversed. Reiki is neither magic nor surgery. Reiki is a practice that you can learn to do yourself or you can find a practitioner to give you Reiki to help address your issues. I encourage you to explore what Reiki can do for you.

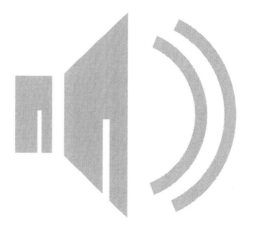

PART FIVE

Raising
Awareness and
Effecting Change

CHAPTER 54
Bring about PD Awareness

"You can't stay in your corner of the Forest waiting for others to come to you. You have to go to them sometimes."—A.A. Milne, *Winnie the Pooh*

Y ou are not your disease. You can, however, be an ambassador of your disease, if you choose to be. Wherever you go, you may educate the public about your condition. Personally, I feel strongly that it is time to educate our communities, the government, and yes, even doctors, about Parkinson's disease. It is time to dispel the many myths that have developed.

Here are four myths we need to dispel.

Myth 1: Only the elderly (and Michael J. Fox) get Parkinson's disease. Well, I'm living proof that this is not true. I got diagnosed with PD in my twenties and so did the many people I meet at the Young-onset Parkinson's conferences. If doctors had known this, it might not have taken six years for them to diagnose me. Michael got diagnosed with PD very young as well.

Most people associate PD with people in their sixties and seventies, but more neurologists are finally recognizing that younger people get PD and it is not just a disease for older people.

Myth 2: There are one million people in the United States with Parkinson's disease. The truth is we actually don't know how many people in the U.S. or any other country in the world have this illness because there is no registry or way of keeping track yet of who has PD.

For more information on the development of a registry or to find out how you can help promote the registry, contact the Parkinson's Action Network (see the Resources section) and your state representatives.

Myth 3: Having deep brain stimulation (DBS) means that the recipient no longer needs to take medication. Not true. DBS is neither a cure for Parkinson's, nor does it mean that you will be able to stop taking your medications. You may need less meds or find that you need to take them less frequently after DBS, but you will probably be on some sort of drug regimen. DBS doesn't end PD, although it has been shown to lessen symptoms and improve the quality of life for some Parkinsonians.

Myth 4: People move uncontrollably and rapidly, or experience dyskinesia, as a symptom of their Parkinson's disease. My understanding is that dyskinesia is not a symptom of the illness directly but comes from too much dopamine being released into the brain at one time. A rapid, explosive, and uncontrollable movement erupts from the dopamine being released, which means it is actually a side effect of medication to treat Parkinson's. Often, if you can lower the potency of a certain med or reduce the frequency with which you take it, your dyskinesia may be lessened.

Ask your doctor before you make any changes, please!

CHAPTER 55
Advocacy Can Lead to Change

"If my mind can conceive it, and my heart can believe it, then I can achieve it."—Muhammad Ali

Each of us has a role to play and a call to action. If we expect change in the field of medicine, our voices need to be heard by those in government, the drug companies, and the insurance industry, as well as physicians and hospital administrators. The future good health of our aging population depends upon finding better solutions to our growing health problems. Better funding and taking a novel look at the science of neurological disorders could lead to major breakthroughs. Sadly, science is dictated by money and it is this reliance on funding that delays the answers from coming.

The brain is still a mystery to us. Little is known about how emotions change our body and our brain. Get involved. Empower yourself and others to make change.

CHAPTER 56
Just Passing Through

There's so much I want to see and do.
Time is limited and I'm just passing through.

I want so much to learn and discover something new.
The world is my classroom while I'm passing through.

Enjoy the stars and sun, snow and sand, and ocean of blue.
Preserve the joys of nature while you're passing through.

The planet was never ours to take; we didn't have a clue.
Cherish life for everything while you're passing through.

The journey is as important as the destination;
stop to see the view.
Savor what you can, because we're all just passing
through.

CHAPTER 57
What Does a "Cure" Mean?

We all seek inner peace. Some of us need the outer too.

What does a cure mean to you? Does it mean stopping the illness where it is or does it mean a complete elimination of the illness totally and completely?

These questions are not easily answered and are a puzzle for patients, researchers, doctors, and most of the rest of those involved in the Parkinson's disease community. I have pondered the question for some time now and think I may have a realistic idea of what may be a fair idea of a cure. My perception of a cure, at this stage of my life, is a treatment or medication that halts disease progression and at least minimizes symptoms of illness with no side effects or bodily harm.

To this date, the closest anything has come to

curing me is a combination of Reiki, yoga, meditation, a vegetarian diet, medication management, and reducing my stress. Together, these factors are having a powerful positive impact on my body. It has taken me years to find what works for me. I hope you find what works for you faster.

I believe that we each must find what works best for ourselves (while avoiding anything harmful) through self-discovery and with the help of our doctors. What works for some, may not work for others. We are all unique and different. Keep an open mind. I'd like to think that we can all find the "cure" that we seek.

?

CHAPTER 58
We Need a Cure

"Every individual makes a difference. We cannot live through a single day without making an impact on the world around us. And we all have free choice—what sort of difference do we want to make? Do we want to make the world around us a better place? Or not?"—Jane Goodall

Doing what is right isn't always easy. It's not popular and sometimes it may be misunderstood. I am not a scientist, but I do know that not long ago brain and heart surgery and organ donation were considered taboo. I would categorize these life-giving procedures as monumental leaps in the right direction. These medical procedures now have saved millions. In the past seventy-five years, modern medicine has gone from thinking that hands should not touch the human heart to discovering DNA and mapping the human genome. Many of the people that I love are still here because of these relatively new and innovative medical procedures.

As one of the over one million people in the United States known to be living with Parkinson's disease, I have been waiting for a cure for over twenty years. American innovation is what made this country a world leader. As someone with young-onset Parkinson's, I am fortunate that the progression of this disease has been slow for me. Since my teens, I have nonetheless watched my balance, speech, coordination, agility, and gait falter due to this illness. I have watched friends divorce, get hospitalized, and die as a result of Parkinson's. If there had been a cure, much of their suffering could have been avoided.

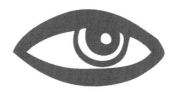

CHAPTER 59
A Surge of Urgency for Parkinson's Disease Treatments and Cure

As a unified group, our community can rally its influence for the causes of better drugs, new therapies, better dissemination of information, and in time, hopefully put an end to Parkinson's disease.

Illness isn't a partisan issue. People on both sides of the aisle in Congress are subject to health problems. People from both sides of our political system are going to need more and better healthcare. Illness doesn't care about socio-economic status, race, or anything else. It has but one mission: to disrupt and challenge people. Life is challenging enough without illness, but when illness combines with everyday existence, life can seem overwhelming.

Lately, there has been talk by politicians and the media about colonizing the Moon. Only in a comedy club would this even be funny! I am a huge NASA fan and fully support a space program. Let's be rational. The technological costs and manpower to perform an operation like this would not only take an astronomical cost, it would also require years of preparation to accomplish this goal, and for what purpose?

For over twenty years, I have been told that in five years we are going to have a cure for Parkinson's disease. I heard this from renowned neurologists and former leaders in the Parkinson's community. They assured me that a cure was in the pipeline. I was, and remain, skeptically hopeful. Until the cure comes, it is up to us, as patients, to do what we can for ourselves.

The United States put a man on the Moon, largely to prove our abilities to the Russians during the Cold War. The important thing to me is that we did it, and in a very short time period. It is this kind of focus and dedication to achievement that is needed to make a breakthrough in curing Parkinson's disease and many other illnesses.

Neurological disorders may be time sensitive, so time is critical. There ought to be a sense of urgency to uncovering the mysteries of illness on this planet before we go colonize Mars, the Moon, or anywhere else in the known universe.

A collective group and a unified voice can encourage change. Advocates for any illness need to make our voices loud if we want to be heard! Staying in touch with the issues and making yourself known to your state and federal representatives is an empowering and proactive way to start becoming an advocate. Work with your local disease organization to stay informed about new and important developments. I encourage you to go to Capitol Hill and walk the halls of Congress for the issues that are important to you.

If you are unable to get to D.C., you can always meet with your representatives in your local district. Change begins with you. With your help, we can encourage more funding and better therapies for the future.

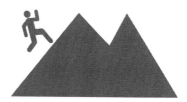

Conclusion

"Don't count the days, make the days count."
—Muhammad Ali

I must restate that you are in control of your own health. If at all possible, you'll want to assemble a medical team of specialists: physicians, a movement disorders specialist, speech pathologists, physical therapists, and practitioners of complementary therapies. You'll also need to get regular exercise, mental stimulation, good nutrition, and most of all lower the stress in your life wherever it exists. Finding patience and erasing negativity will serve you well. If the mind remains positive, the body is more likely to take on the message to heal.

We owe it to ourselves and those we care about to be as healthy as we possibly can. Exploring unconventional, non-invasive complementary therapies like massage, cranial sacral, reiki, qigong, and whatever else calls to you, is worth it. Be openly skeptical and hopeful. When I was first introduced to reiki, I was neither open nor particularly hopeful. Only through trying the actual energy work was I able to overcome my skepticism about its efficacy. Each of our journeys is unique and therefore calls for different combinations of medicine and therapy. I truly believe that with an open mind, a positive attitude, working with doctors, maintaining a beneficial diet and exercise regimen, calming the mind, and exploring complementary therapies, we can experience positive changes in our lives. The more we are able to listen to our bodies and calm our minds, the better our whole mental-emotional-spiritual-physical system will be. I wish you the very best on your journey for answers and hope that you discover what works for you. Finding what works will take dedication and perseverance, but it very well may direct you on your path to healing.

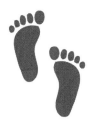

FINAL INSIGHTS
A Few of the Lessons I've Learned from Parkinson's Disease

"Our greatest glory is not in never falling, but in rising every time we fall."—Confucius (551–479 B.C.E.)

- You have a choice how you treat yourself and others. Starting the day with a smile and a positive perspective brightens your day and those you encounter.
- Plan as much as you can, but remain flexible and be prepared for changes. Book some events, such as outings, a backyard picnic, a game night, a favorite movie, or a favorite meal, so you always have something to look

forward to, and yet be willing to alter these plans as needed.

- Set realistic goals that will give you a sense of accomplishment. Start small and work your way up. Have a plan and a goal to work toward.
- Don't be too hard on yourself when you falter. Everyone has tough days.
- Keep inspired. Amazing events are happening all around us all the time. See the morning sunrise. Watch the night sky. Observe. Appreciate.
- Help a total stranger in any way you can, just for the sake of helping. See what happens.
- Eat organic produce, if you can. I know PD patients who gave up artificial sweeteners or certain processed foods and found they felt better and experienced reduced symptoms. Going gluten-free may be an option to consider.
- Avoid shrimp, clams, mollusks, and most seafood, as these creatures filter seawater, and thus their bodies collect the toxins in our oceans.
- Eat as low on the food chain as you can—meaning, eat as many plants as possible. I have observed how protein interferes with the efficacy of my medication. Try an experiment: Cut out meat for a few days to see and feel the difference. Notice if this improves your energy and helps your skin. Animal flesh can accumulate toxins, depending upon what it is fed.
- Avoid MAO inhibitor "trigger" drugs, like cold and flu medications, as these can cause serious interactions. Read drug warning labels.
- Explore the role stress plays in your life and seek ways to address it. Stress reduces the

effectiveness of meds, disturbs sleep, and can cause more illnesses. Try speaking with a friend, therapist, or a counselor. Find an outlet for stress, like calming your mind through yoga, exercise, Reiki, and meditation.

- Don't ignore your physical health and stamina. Stay physically active as best you can. Play a Nintendo Wii, walk, look at the advice in John Argue's book and video *Parkinson's Disease and the Art of Moving* (New Harbinger Publications, 2000).
- Stay informed about developments in Parkinson's disease medicine and technology.
- Empower yourself and get involved, whether it is through advocacy in the Parkinson's Action Network (PAN) or fundraising for National Parkinson Foundation (NPF), American Parkinson Disease Association (APDA), Parkinson Disease Foundation (PDF), Michael J. Fox Foundation, Parkinson Alliance (Unity Walk), or The Parkinson's Institute and Clinical Center.
- Find a support group in your area. Contact the NPF, the APDA, and PDF for more information about updates and seminars. Visit their websites (see Resources).
- Eat high-fiber foods like prunes, grains, and apples.
- Stay hydrated. Drink water throughout the day to avoid dehydration and constipation.
- Know your medications! Know when you take them, why you take them, and what types of potential side effects could occur. Read the package inserts that come with your medications, and speak with your doctor or pharma-

cist if you have questions or concerns.
- Stay active: Be it with yoga, walking, weights, or swimming—just do something.
- If your speech needs help, look into finding a certified LSVT clinician. Look into SPEAK-OUT® voice program provided by Parkinson Voice Project (see Resources).
- Consider improving your digestion with a probiotic supplement.
- Keep your mind active and challenged.
- Avoid potent cleaning supplies, air fresheners, processed foods, and artificial odor products like cheap candles with infused odors that may cause headaches or worse. Look for natural essential oils. Young Living Essential Oils are especially good.
- Search for a neurologist with whom you can communicate. Find a neurologist who is also a movement disorders specialist, if possible.
- Sleep matters. You need rest to recharge those dopamine receptors. If you can't sleep, talk to your doctor.
- Keep active. Challenge your mind and body daily. Try puzzles. But don't overdo it—find a balance.
- Stay on track. Keep a schedule with your meds and take them on time with water.
- Music can soothe headaches, improve mood, and help you to relax.
- Stay informed. Sign up to get Google alerts about local chapters of PD organizations and other legitimate PD sites to get the latest press on Parkinson's disease.
- Forgive the person who cut you off or took

your parking spot. Let insensitive comments go, even if they hurt you. Rise above hurtful talk and poor behavior—just let it vaporize.

- Tell the people in your life how much they mean to you. Do something unexpected, like coming home from work early to play with your kids, taking your spouse out for lunch, or doing something as simple as writing a love poem and offering a hug.
- Call a friend you think of often yet haven't spoken to for awhile. Don't put it off!
- Do at least three kind deeds a day, anything from complimenting someone, to opening a door for someone, or helping a neighbor with his or her computer troubles.
- Share some helpful knowledge with others, through an email, a post on Facebook, Twitter, a phone call, or in person.
- Give the animals in your life extra affection, play time, and grooming.
- The next time you get angry, try replacing that feeling with compassion for someone else.
- A simple smile can brighten your day and someone else's, too.
- Laugh as much as you can.
- Taking power from someone else hurts you and the person you rob.
- Cynicism, doubt, and ego are anti-social, and contribute to pain, anger, and suffering.
- Negative thinking and negative energy is unhealthy and wasteful. Positive thinking can change the world.
- Time is yours to manage.
- Performing a kind act for disingenuous reasons

has no merit.

- Denial is far easier than acceptance.
- Taking the easy way rarely completes the task at hand in a satisfactory manner.
- Never let illness defeat you. Your will and drive to heal, can and will, overcome PD. Each day brings hope for improvement. Your thoughts are capable of assisting your body to improve from its current state. Do your best to take care of yourself and preserve your health.
- Avoid the trilogy of regret: I should've! I would've! I could've!
- Platinum rule: Do unto others better than they do unto you.
- Be kind to yourself as you face this daunting challenge. Living and battling illness takes grit, perseverance, patience, determination, focus, and a sense of humor.
- Take the time to find the treasures in your life!
- Free yourself of negative influences. Your physician and medical support system should make life easier for you. It is essential to build a support network of your spouse, friends, family, children, animals, social worker, and a medical team.
- Support groups can be a cathartic outlet for your emotions, as well as a wonderful way to meet and learn from others.
- Practice affirmations: "Today is my opportunity to make a difference. Today, I can be the catalyst for initiating change in some small way. Today, I have life and life is not to be wasted. Today is unique from all others. Today, I am alive! Today, I appreciate the ele-

ments of nature and all the beauty that it encompasses. Today, I realize that simple pleasures truly are the very best."

- We humans are adaptable creatures. When forced to survive harsh environmental tests or extreme conditions, we adapt to the task presented upon us. Illness is no different than climbing a mountain. It takes preparation, training, fortitude and pacing yourself for the journey ahead.

- You are a unique individual, but you are not alone. There are lessons in suffering. Illness plays a role in all aspects of life. Don't overlook speaking to those close to you about how they are dealing with your illness. Helping others feel good relieves the burden for both of you.

- Sometimes, when diagnosed with an illness, our motivation changes. Illness can detour or at least alter plans and hopes. We can't plan for all the changes or roadblocks in our life. As your disease changes, so shall your independence. You will be much happier and reduce stress if you learn to accept what you can't change and to be malleable and forgiving.

- You must have a focus that drives you forward. For some of us, that focus is to get better and heal ourselves—or at least slow the progression of illness. Some may want to bring awareness to the world about the disease for which they are afflicted. Some may fight for change or better funding.

- Even in our chaotic world, peace is all around us, just waiting for discovery. Whether it is the harmony of nature in a city center or ducks on a pond, take time to savor nature and truly appreciate the world. Watch how bugs interact and beads of water flow and pool. The calming of nature adds to our peaceful being. Nature's beauty should be part of your day.

- Each day is an opportunity to grow as a human being. Each day is a chance to feel better and to improve your condition. Each day means a time to celebrate and commemorate the gifts of life. Each day means focusing on what you have rather than what you don't.
- Illness can rob you of your dignity, as well as your confidence, if you let it. It is crucial that you keep perspective and know, in your mind and heart, that you are doing your very best to perform at a higher level. You are a survivor.
- Often, when one opportunity dries up, another presents itself. A door closes, but a window opens. One of the biggest lessons of having PD and running a business with Angela has been to have faith in what we are doing.
- When you are feeling poorly or experiencing indecision, it is easy to relinquish too much responsibility to your care partner and/or companion. Be aware of the strain that you both may experience as you both come to accept and share your needs with one another. Your partner is dealing with your illness every day, just as you are. Be sensitive to his or her issues.
- Your partner is dealing with your illness from another perspective, so communication is key. Try to see your PD from your caregiver or care partner's point of view.
- One key to life is identifying what decisions will

truly impact you and which ones won't. A major discovery for me was that there is a right time to relinquish control to others. Sometimes when we give up the tight reigns of control, we can actually feel better and improve our overall health. Pick your battles wisely and realize that you can't control the majority of your life. Some decisions are just out of your control.

- Life is short no matter how long you live. Love what you do and do what you love. When I had an opportunity to work for myself, my dream came true.
- Illness is an opportunity to teach yourself and others! Don't just perceive illness as a battle, fight, or war. Illness is a wakeup call to seeing the world in its entire splendor. Illness teaches compassion, understanding, peace, and harmony, if you let it. You have a choice in how you envision your life. Much of your destiny depends on what you do and the example you set for those around you.
- There is a place for conventional medicine and complementary medicine. You must uncover what works for you. Only through exploration, personal growth, education, and discovery can you proceed with healing. Understand your illness as fully as you can so that you may make the wisest decisions to overcome your ailment.
- Make yourself and your care partner known to your doctors. Doctors are often rushed, stressed, and overwhelmed with work. Ask for what you want from your doctor and if you can't get it, you may have to go to another.
- Your doctor should explain why he or she is

doing what is being done. If you have a problem or question, speak up. The doctor works for you.

- There must be mutual respect between doctor and patient for the relationship to work. Your doctor should know your name. Your doctor should answer questions, listen to you, and be up to date on research. A good bedside manner is a nice plus; however, try to accept that a talented physician may be more important.
- The shock of being diagnosed with a chronic illness is a life-altering experience. Your world doesn't have to be turned upside down. The best thing that you can do is educate yourself and look for advancements in therapies, drugs, medical technologies, and complementary treatments that may show promise. Your life is precious. You fought to enter this world, now fight to stay in it!
- Don't give up on your well-being! Options abound. Be on the lookout for rehab and assistive devices that may have solutions to assist with improving certain qualities of life. These resources may restore, or at least temporarily bring back, abilities you thought were gone for good. There are some solutions out there that you probably never even knew existed. Keep informed about these through websites, newsletters, emails, blogs, forums, and conferences. Go to support groups and share your wisdom with others. Teach, learn, and share what you know.
- If disease brings about any positive illumination in our lives, it is the light of self-discovery. Dis-

ease is a test of knowing yourself. Through the experience of disease, you can learn an appreciation for all aspects of life, both the good and bad. Life is life and while the next one may be even better, you can enjoy this one to its fullest.

- Our lives can change in a moment's notice, whether that is through a dramatic correction in the stock market, a natural disaster, a car wreck, or the onset of illness of a loved one. As much as we would like to believe that we can steer our future, there will always be elements of life that are simply out of our reach. Some beasts are untamable and there are rivers that will swell outside their shores. Sometimes we forget that we are only visitors staying in Hotel Earth and checkout time is when she says so.
- Life should be measured in quality, not quantity.
- Don't lose the passion for the activities and simple pleasures of life. You are limited to a point, but there are solutions. If you can no longer draw, you could transition into photos. Savor music, art, literature, cinema, and stay open-minded. Do not focus on the loss of "what could've been," instead lock in on what you are still capable of doing, enjoying, and achieving.
- Do your best to think and act in a positive and optimistic manner. Today means an opportunity to grow. You have a choice to be okay with who you are and to continue to better yourself and the lives of those around you.
- Appreciate your care partner for making a difference in your quality of life.
- Animals are healing beings. They make you laugh. They share emotions and provide us

with unconditional love, understanding, and companionship.

- Know your medications, options, and your illness. The more you understand your disease, the more options you may have available to you.
- Illness teaches compassion, tolerance, and patience.
- Parkinson's forces one to learn the art of patience whether one chooses it or not.
- PD teaches compassion and understanding for others.
- Make the most of your good days and maximize your better days.
- Push your limits, but know your limitations.
- If you are in public and are stared at because of your illness, this is a prime opportunity to be an ambassador of education for your illness.
- A hopeful attitude makes life better.
- Focus on what you are still capable of doing.
- Keep a flexible schedule to reduce your stress level.
- Never blame yourself.
- Learn as much as you can about available therapies.
- Helping others helps you.
- Say thank you to your caregiver, carepartner, family, friends, medical team, and anyone else that helps you. It is important that you acknowledge their contributions to your life and health.

Recommended Resources

Here are some helpful organizations, websites/blogs, and books to offer you additional information and support. As resources are always changing, please view an up-to-date listing at ASoftVoice.com.

PARKINSON'S DISEASE ORGANIZATIONS
There are organizations all over the world that support the Parkinson's community. Here are listings for the United States, Canada, and the United Kingdom.

American Parkinson Disease Association (APDA)
APDAParkinson.org
800-223-2732
Maintains support group and information chapters all over the country. Also started the National Young Onset Center, providing information to those living with young-onset PD, YoungParkinsons.org.

Davis Phinney Foundation for Parkinson's
DavisPhinneyFoundation.org
To provide inspiration, practical tools and information to help people live well with Parkinson's. Hosts The Victory Summit® held around the country to inspire those living with PD and their loved ones, publishes The Every Victory Counts® program manual, and holds Living Well Challenge® webinars.

NPF Georgia
NPFGeorgia.org
This organization has a large network of support groups for those with Parkinson's and their caregivers/care partners. Hosts the Southeastern Parkinson Disease Conference every fall in Atlanta.

Michael J. Fox Foundation for Parkinson's Research
MichaelJFox.org
800-708-7644
The Michael J. Fox Foundation is dedicated to finding a cure for Parkinson's disease through an aggressively funded research agenda and to ensuring the development of improved therapies for those living with Parkinson's today. Fox Trial Finder is a way for people to sign up and participate in clinical trial research.

Movers & Shakers
PDOutreach.org
A national organization that promotes outreach and advocacy to the Parkinson's community. Started by a wife and husband who both have PD.

National PD Research Education Clinical Center (PA-DRECC) and Veterans Affairs PD Consortium (VAPD)
Parkinsons.VA.gov
Six specialized Centers of Excellence created by the Department of Veteran Affairs created to serve the estimated 80,000 veterans affected by PD through state-of-the-art clinical care, education, research, and national outreach and advocacy.

National Parkinson Foundation (NPF)
Parkinson.org
800-473-4636
NPF has a national network of support groups, publishes free educational manuals covering PD topics, and in partnership with the APDA, hosts the Young Onset Parkinson Conferences. NPF also has a program to certify Centers of Excellence in Parkinson's disease care to designate outstanding providers of Parkinson's care.

Northwest Parkinson's Foundation (NWPF)
NWPF.org
877-980-7500
NWPF is a nonprofit organization established to improve quality of life for the northwest Parkinson's disease community. NWPF has the Booth Gardner Parkinson's Care Center in Kirkland, Washington; Parkinson's TeleHealth Program; caregiver training; and support groups.

Parkinson's Action Network (PAN)
ParkinsonsAction.org
800-850-4726
PAN serves as the unified voice of the Parkinson's

community advocating for better treatments and a cure. In partnership with other Parkinson's organizations and our powerful grassroots network, we educate the public and government leaders on better policies for research and an improved quality of life for people living with Parkinson's. PAN is a grassroots organization that empowers the PD community to advocate for issues affecting our community.

Parkinson Alliance/Parkinson's Unity Walk

ParkinsonAlliance.org
800-579-8440
The Parkinson Alliance is a national nonprofit organization in partnership with The Tuchman Foundation, dedicated to raising funds to help finance promising PD research. They host the Parkinson's Unity Walk each year in New York City. The Alliance is also dedicated to improving the quality of life in the DBS community.

Parkinson's Disease Foundation (PDF)

PDF.org
800-457-6676
PDF provides many online and printed materials on PD, publishes Parkinson's Disease Resource List, hosts many webcasts and teleseminars, trains those with PD to become research advocates to learn more about PD research, hosts events all over the country, and encourages creativity by creating the annual Creativity and Parkinson's calendar.

Parkinson Foundation of the National Capital Area (PFNCA)

ParkinsonFoundation.org

PFNCA strives to provide education and support to people in Virginia, Maryland, and the District of Columbia through a large network of support groups and exercise, dance, and choir programs.. Holds an annual regional symposium.

Parkinson Society of Canada (PSC)

Parkinson.Ca

800-565-3000

PSC is the national voice of Canadians living with Parkinson's. It provides education, support services, advocacy, and funding for research on behalf of over 100,000 Canadians coping with this brain disease every day.

Parkinson's UK

Parkinsons.org.UK

0808-800-0303

Provides a support group network, publications, and a free confidential helpline for those living with PD in the United Kingdom. Also sponsors many events each year, including Moving Forward Together, an event for younger people affected by Parkinson's.

Parkinson Voice Project

ParkinsonVoiceProject.org

855-707-7325

Parkinson Voice Project is to preserve the voices of individuals with Parkinson's and related neurological disorders through intensive voice therapy, follow up support, research, education, and community awareness. All who need treatment receive it free through a "Pay it Forward" model.

YOUNG ONSET RESOURCES

American Parkinson Disease Association National Young Onset Center
YoungParkinsons.org
877-223-3801
The ADPA National Young Onset Center focuses on developing education and support services that address the unique needs of young people with Parkinson's disease, their family members and friends, as well as their healthcare team.

APDA Young Parkinson's Handbook
StLaPDA.org
Search for this free handbook under their "Downloads" menu. It is a guide for young Parkinson's patients and their families.

PD BLOGS, WEBSITES, ONLINE SUPPORT
Websites and blogs written by those living with Parkinson's disease.

A Soft Voice in a Noisy World
ASoftVoice.com
In my blog, I share my medical journey with readers, and encourage them to seek all avenues that can benefit their condition.

BrainTalk Communities

BrainTalkCommunities.org
BrainTalk Communities is a listing of online patient support groups for neurology.

Parkinson's Humor

ParkinsonsHumor.Blogspot.com
Bev Ribaudo, aka YumaBev, fights Parkinson's by laughing and sharing her insights with the world.

Patients Like Me

PatientsLikeMe.com
A website to share your real world health experiences to help yourself, other patients like you, and the healthcare community. On this site you can create your own blog and/or meet other bloggers.

PDPlan4Life

PDPlan4Life.com
Written by Jean and Sheryl, who are living with Parkinson's disease. They share their journeys along with providing wonderful tips about living well with PD.

CONFERENCES

Conferences and symposia are great ways to connect with others living with PD who are in your area, and to also learn about the latest news in treatments and research. Check with your local or regional PD organization to find ones near you.

Davis Phinney Foundation/The Victory Summit®

DavisPhinneyFoundation.org/victory-summit/up-coming-victory-summits/

The Victory Summit® Symposia Series occurs around the country each year to inspire and motivate those living with Parkinson's to live well.

Southeastern Parkinson Disease Conference

NPFGeorgia.org

This annual regional conference brings in speakers from all over the country speaking on a variety of topics. The conference also highlights speakers who are living with Parkinson's disease.

World Parkinson Congress

WorldPDCongress.org

The World Parkinson Congresses provide an international forum for the latest scientific discoveries, medical practices and care initiatives related to Parkinson disease. By bringing physicians, scientists, nurses, rehab professionals, policy advocates, care partners, family members and people with Parkinson's disease together, we aim to create a worldwide dialogue that will help expedite the discovery of a cure and best treatment practices for this devastating disease.

Young Onset Parkinson Conferences

Parkinson.org/Improving-Care/Education/Education--For-Patients/Young-Onset-Conferences

The American Parkinson Disease Association National Young-Onset Center and the National Parkinson Foundation have partnered up to offer regional conference for those living with young-onset Parkinson's and their loved ones. This conference provides up-to-date information on research, treatments, and living well with PD.

PARKINSON'S DISEASE BOOKS
A short listing of the many books about living with Parkinson's.

Delay the Disease: Exercise and PD by David Zid, A.C.E., A.C.G., and Jackie Russell, R.N., B.S.N., C.N.O.R. David Zid, 2007.

HOPE: Four Keys to a Better Quality of Life for Parkinson's People by Hal Newsom. Mercer Island, WA.: The Northwest Parkinson's Foundation, 2002.

Living Well, Running Hard: Lessons Learned from Living with Parkinson's Disease by John Ball. iUniverse.com, 2011.

Living Well with Parkinson's Disease: What Your Doctor Doesn't Tell You...that You Need to Know by Michael J. Church and Gretchen Garie. New York, N.Y.: HarperCollins Publishers, 2012.

Life with a Battery-Operated Brain: A Patient's Guide to Deep Brain Stimulation Surgery for Parkinson's Disease by Jackie Hunt Christiensen. Minneapolis, MN.: Langdon Street Press, 2009.

Making the Connection Between Brain and Behavior: Coping with Parkinson's Disease by Joseph H. Friedman. New York, N.Y.: Demos Medical Publishing, 2008.

Parkinson's Disease: A Complete Guide for Patients and Families, Second Edition by Anthony E. Lang, Lisa M. Schulman, and William J. Weiner. Baltimore, MD.: The John's Hopkins University Press, 2007.

Parkinson's Disease and the Art of Moving by John Argue. Oakland, CA.: New Harbinger Publications, 2000.

Saving Milly: Love, Politics, and Parkinson's Disease by Morton Kondracke. New York, N.Y.: Ballantine Books, 2002.

Surviving Adversity: Living with Parkinson's Disease by Gord Carley. Toronto, Canada: Surviving Adversity, 2007.

The First Year—Parkinson's Disease: An Essential Guide for the Newly Diagnosed by Jackie Hunt Christiensen. New York, N.Y.: Marlowe & Company, 2005.

What's Shakin': An Insider's Look at the Humorous Side of Parkinson's Disease by John Brissette. Lincoln, NE.: iUniverse, 2007.

What Your Doctor May Not Tell You about Parkinson's Disease: A Holistic Program for Optimal Wellness by Jill Marjama-Lyons. New York, N.Y.: Warner Books, 2003.

ADDITIONAL BOOKS
These are books mentioned in *A Soft Voice*, along with others that may be of interest.

A Path with Heart: A Guide Through the Perils and Promises of Spiritual Life by Jack Kornfield. New York, N.Y.: Bantam Books, 1993.

Mindfulness in Plain English by Venerable Henepola Guaratano. Somerville, MA.: Wisdom Publications, 2002.

Wherever You Go, There You Are: Mindfulness Meditation in Everyday Life by Jon Kabat-Zinn. New York, N.Y.: Hyperion, 2005.

Full Catastrophe Living: Using the Wisdom of Your Body and Mind to Face Stress, Pain, and Illness by Jon Kabat-Zinn. New York: N.Y.: Delta Trade Paperbacks, 1991.

Coming to Our Senses: Healing Ourselves and the World Through Mindfulness by Jon Kabat-Zinn. New York, N.Y.: Hyperion, 2006.

You Can Heal Your Life by Louise Hay. Carlsbad, CA.: Hay House, 2007.

PARKINSON'S MAGAZINES AND NEWSLETTERS
Many of the national and international PD organizations provide free paper and electronic newsletters for the PD community.

Neurology Now
Neurologynow.com
Neurology Now, a free bimonthly online and print publication of the American Academy of Neurology, provides patients and their caregivers with credible, up-to-the-minute, balanced coverage of the latest advances in neurology research and treatment.

Parkinson's Disease Foundation
PDF.org/en/pdf_newsletter

PARKINSON'S DOCUMENTARIES

10 Mountains 10 Years, directed by Jennifer Yee (Back Light Productions LLC, 2011)

FRONTLINE: My Father, My Brother & Me, written and directed by Dave Iverson (PBS Home Video, 2009).

Shaken: Journey into the Mind of a Parkinson's Patient, written and directed by Deborah J. Fryer (Lila Films, 2007).

ADDITIONAL PARKINSON'S RESOURCES

The following websites may help you to take action on the ideas you've been reading about in this book. Although this is by no means a complete list of resources for people living with Parkinson's disease and their care partners, I hope these will be useful and informative.

MEDICAL INFORMATION SITES

Mayo Clinic
MayoClinic.com
The Mayo Clinic can help you find information on hundreds of conditions. You can also check your symptoms and get help discovering ways to improve your lifestyle. The Mayo Clinic can also diagnose and treat your condition.

MedlinePlus
MedlinePlus.gov
MedlinePlus is the National Institutes of Health's website designed for consumers. Produced by the National Library of Medicine, it offers information about diseases, conditions, and wellness issues in understandable language. You can use MedlinePlus to learn about the latest treatments, look up information on a drug or a nutritional supplement, find out the meanings of medical words, or view medical videos or illustrations. You can also get links to the latest medical research on your topic, or find out about clinical trials on a disease or condition.

Parkinson's Information Exchange Network
Parkinsons-Information-Exchange-Network-Online.com
This exchange network lets to see archived information about Parkinson's disease, including access to an answer center, an email support list, a drug database, current topics related to Parkinson's, and much more.

PubMed
NCBI.NLM.NIH.gov/pubmed
You can use PubMed to access millions of available searches of the National Library of Medicine and databases. PubMed comprises more than twenty-one million citations for biomedical literature from Medline, life science journals, and online books. Citations may include links to full-text content from PubMed Central and publisher websites.

WebMD
WebMD.com
WebMD provides valuable health information, tools for managing your health, and support to those who seek information. You can trust that their content is timely and credible.

WE MOVE™
WEMOVE.org
WE MOVE™ is a not-for-profit organization that utilizes creativity, innovation, and collaborative approaches to improve awareness, diagnosis, and management of movement disorders among people living with these conditions and the professionals who care for them.

RESEARCH AND MEDICAL TRIALS
Participating in clinical trials is a way to help advance scientific research in Parkinson's.

23andMe
www.23andMe.com/pd/
Help revolutionize the way Parkinson's disease is

studied and accelerate the search for a cure. Take an active role in groundbreaking research by mailing in your DNA sample and answering surveys online. Over 6,500 people with Parkinson's have come together to form what is now the largest Parkinson's community for genetic research in the world.

Fox Trial Finder
FoxTrialFinder.MichaelJFox.org
Register to find out what trials are in your area and information about clinical trials you may qualify for.

National Institute of Neurological Disorders and Stroke
NINDS.NIH.gov/research/parkinsonsweb/index. htm
This part of the NINDS website gives an overview of Parkinson's disease research.

Parkinson Pipeline Project
PDPipeline.org
A group of volunteers with Parkinson's who are committed to providing the patient's perspective in the treatment development process.

WELLNESS, EXERCISE, AND MOVEMENT

Delay the Disease
DelaytheDisease.com
Founded by David Zid, Delay the Disease is a Parkinson's specific exercise program based on the latest scientific research. Find books, videos, and

support on the website.

International Sheng Zhen Society

ShengZhen.org
Master Li's teachings in Sheng Zhen Healing Qigong can be practiced by anyone and is helpful to
those living with illness.

LSVT Global (Lee Silverman Voice Treatment)

LSVT.org
LSVT Global pioneered the Lee Silverman Voice
Treatment (LSVT), an innovative and clinically
proven method for improving voice and speech in
individuals with Parkinson's disease. Today, LSVT
specializes in the development of innovative and
effective treatments for the speech communication (LSVT LOUD) and physical/occupational therapy (LSVT BIG) needs of individuals with Parkinson's disease.

Mindfulness Meditation with Jon Kabat-Zinn

MindfulnessTapes.com
A series of stress reduction and meditation tapes
to help users experience the universal aspects of
stillness and well-being, clarity, wisdom, compassion, and self-compassion without the ideological
or cultural trappings that so often make it difficult
for Westerners to experience medication.

Reiki

ReikiJinKeiDo.org
This website provides information about Reiki and
gives a list of Reiki masters. For a legitimate Reiki master, I don't advise working with someone

who received Reiki mastership training in a single weekend.

Parkinson's Disease and The Art of Moving
ParkinsonsExercise.com
These exercises are focused directly on Parkinson's symptoms. You can do the exercises at your own pace, either from the book or DVD that they produced.

Rock Steady Boxing
RockSteadyBoxing.org
Scott C. Newman, who is living with early-onset Parkinson's, founded rock Steady Boxing, the first and only boxing program of its kind in the country, in 2006. The seed for what would eventually become the Rock Steady Boxing Foundation was planted when Newman began intense, one-on-one boxing training with friend just a few years after he was diagnosed. Newman's quality of life improved dramatically in a short time due to his fighting back against Parkinson's disease.

RESEARCHING YOUR DOCTOR: DO YOU KNOW YOUR DOCTOR?
Most of us spend more time researching a new car or a new major appliance than we do our doctors. You entrust your health to someone you may know almost nothing about. You may have a doctor simply because he or she is assigned to you by your provider. If you have Parkinson's disease and your neurologist isn't a "movement disorder specialist," you may want to find one who is. Who you choose

for your doctor is a matter of choice, of course; but keep in mind that a specialist concentrates on helping PD patient's movements. Here are some resources that can help you research doctors and choose ones that are best for you.

American Board of Medical Specialties
www.ABMS.org
ABMS is focused on improving the safety and quality of medical care by working with our member boards to set the standards for physician specialty certification and continuous education. Part of this focus involves providing products and services for public and professional use to verify physician board certification.

Administrators in Medicine
DocBoard.org
Administrators in Medicine, a not-for-profit organization, is the national organization for state medical and osteopathic board executives. Founded in 1984, the mission of AIM is to assist and support administrators for medical licensing and regulatory authorities to achieve administrative excellence and ultimately advance public safety. Services offered include educational, research, and online services for its members.

Angie's List
AngiesList.com
A word-of-mouth network for consumers, Angie's List is a growing collection of homeowners' real-life experiences with local service companies. The people who join Angie's List are like you: look-

ing for a way to find trustworthy companies that perform high-quality work.

Consumers' Checkbook
Checkbook.org
Consumers' Checkbook, The Center for the Study of Services, is an independent, nonprofit consumer organization founded in 1974 with the help of funding from the U.S. Office of Consumer Affairs. Their purpose is to provide consumers information to help them get high-quality services and products at the best possible prices.

Directory of State Medical and Osteopathic Boards
FSMB.org/directory_smb.html
A complete listing of contact information for medical and osteopathic boards by state.

DocInfo
www.DocInfo.org
The Federation of State Medical Boards has collected data on physicians for more than forty years. Available to the public is the FSMB Physician Profile from their comprehensive, nationally consolidated data bank of U.S. licensed physicians. The FSMB Physician Profile provides professional information on medical doctors, osteopathic physicians, and the majority of physician assistants licensed in the U.S. They not only search the state where the physician is currently practicing, they also search all known practice locations throughout the U.S.

Families USA
FamiliesUSA.org
Families USA is a national nonprofit, non-partisan organization dedicated to the achievement of high-quality, affordable health care for all Americans. Working at the national, state, and community levels, they have earned a national reputation as an effective voice for health care consumers for twenty-five years.

HealthGrades
HealthGrades.com
HealthGrades has become the way 200 million consumers look for a new physician or hospital and their Patient Direct Connect product is fast becoming the way hospitals connect with consumers to find, evaluate, select, and connect with a physician online.

Health Resources and Services Administration
HRSA.gov
The Health Resources and Services Administration, an agency of the U.S. Department of Health and Human Services, is the primary federal agency for improving access to health care services for people who are uninsured, isolated or medically vulnerable.

Hospital-Data
Hospital-Data.com
The Hospital-Data site will help you to research hospitals and nursing homes online. They have profiles of thousands of hospitals, medical clinics, and nursing homes.

MyDocHub

MyDocHub.com

MyDocHub is an online health community for you and your friends to anonymously review and rate your doctor experience on punctuality, waiting room times, total time spent in the office, and staff efficiency. Also, you will be able to share your health-related videos and participate on their health forums and blog.

Rate MD's

RateMDs.com

Use this website to browse reviews of over one million doctors.

UCompare Health Care

UCompareHealthCare.com

UCompare Health Care helps people make better decisions about their healthcare choices. Their free reports help you find, research, and compare hospitals, nursing homes, doctors, fertility centers, and mammography centers.

Vitals

Vitals.com

Vitals was created to give consumers the tools to make informed decisions about which doctor to choose. The website offers a variety of ways to find a doctor that's right for you.

HELPFUL WEBSITES AND ASSISTIVE TOOLS

Aids for Arthritis
AidsforArthritis.com
Founded in 1979, Aids for Arthritis is the oldest and largest arthritis self-help products company in the United States. Their products are selected by medical professionals to promote joint preservation and energy conservation, and to reduce pain.

Allsup
Allsup.com
Allsup has been helping people obtain Social Security disability insurance (SSDI) awards nationwide for twenty-five years with a 98 percent success rate.

Aware in Care Kit
AwareinCare.org
Kit contains a hospital action plan book on how to plan for a hospital visit, a Parkinson's ID bracelet, a medical alert card, a medication form, a PD fact sheet for medical professionals, and more.

Canine Assistants for Parkinson's
CanineAssistants.org
Canine Assistants is a non-profit organization, which trains and provides service dogs for children and adults with physical disabilities or other special needs.

Closing the Gap
ClosingtheGap.com
Closing the Gap provides assistive technology re-

sources and training opportunities through its bi-monthly (print and online) magazine, webinars, and annual international conference. It is a comprehensive guide to assistive technology and devices.

Create Your Own Parkinson's Medical Alert Card
Nuppy.net/MedAlert/php/MedCardForm.php
This website (very well done by my friend, Brian!) allows you to create your own Parkinson's disease medical alert card, which includes your personal information as well as a listing of the medications you use, including dosages and frequency.

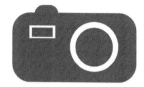

About the Author

Karl Robb has had Parkinson's disease (PD) for over twenty years. With symptoms since he was seventeen years old, Karl was diagnosed at the age of twenty-three. Now in his forties, he is a Parkinson's advocate, an entrepreneur, an inventor, a writer, a speaker on PD issues, a photographer, and a Reiki master.

Karl holds a bachelor's degree in English from the University of North Carolina at Chapel Hill. His work on PD issues has been featured by *The New York Post,* BBC Radio, the CBS News, and NHK World Television, as well as several Washington, D.C., television stations.

Karl is a board member and the Virginia state director of the Parkinson's Action Network and a board member of the Parkinson Voice Project.

To contact Karl, email him at karl@asoftvoice.com.